COGNITIVE-BEHAVIORAL THERAPIES
WITH LESBIAN, GAY, AND BISEXUAL CLIENTS

Cognitive-Behavioral Therapies with Lesbian, Gay, and Bisexual Clients

CHRISTOPHER R. MARTELL
STEVEN A. SAFREN
STACEY E. PRINCE

Foreword by Marvin R. Goldfried

THE GUILFORD PRESS
New York   London

© 2004 The Guilford Press
A Division of Guilford Publications, Inc.
72 Spring Street, New York, NY 10012
www.guilford.com

Printed in the United States of America

This book is printed on acid-free paper.

Last digit is print number: 9 8 7 6 5 4 3 2 1

Library of Congress Cataloging-in-Publication Data

Martell, Christopher R.
  Cognitive-behavioral therapies with lesbian, gay, and bisexual clients
/ Christopher R. Martell, Steven A. Safren, Stacey E. Prince ; foreword
by Marvin R. Goldfried.
       p. cm.
Includes bibliographical references and index.
  ISBN 1-57230-954-7 (hbk. : alk. paper)
  1. Lesbians—Mental health. 2. Gays—Mental health. 3.
Bisexuals—Mental health. 4. Lesbians—Counseling of. 5.
Gays—Counseling of. 6. Bisexuals—Counseling of. 7. Cognitive
therapy. I. Safren, Steven A. II. Prince, Stacey Ellen. III. Title.
  RC451.4.G39M37 2004
  616.89'142'08664—dc22

                                              2003017548

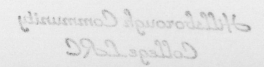

About the Authors

Christopher R. Martell, PhD, maintains a private practice in Seattle and is Clinical Associate Professor of Psychology at the University of Washington. He serves as a member of the American Psychological Association's Committee on Lesbian, Gay, and Bisexual Concerns, and is a past president of the Washington State Psychological Association. In addition, Dr. Martell is board certified in both clinical psychology and behavioral psychology through the American Board of Professional Psychology and is a founding fellow of the Academy of Cognitive Therapy. A coauthor (with Michael Addis and the late Neil Jacobson) of *Depression in Context: Strategies for Guided Action,* he has published articles and book chapters on behavioral treatments for depression and issues affecting gay, lesbian, and bisexual individuals.

Steven A. Safren, PhD, is Assistant Professor of Psychology at Harvard Medical School, Associate Director of the Cognitive-Behavioral Therapy Program at Massachusetts General Hospital, and a research scientist at Fenway Community Health, an urban health center that primarily serves the lesbian, gay, bisexual, and transgendered (LGBT) community. Dr. Safren is actively involved in clinical research, and has published in the areas of LGBT mental health, behavioral aspects of HIV and cognitive-behavioral approaches to HIV medication adherence, and mood and anxiety disorders. At Massachusetts General Hospital, he also teaches and supervises psychology interns and medical residents in cognitive-behavioral therapy, and is currently the Principal Investigator of a National Institute of Mental Health-funded study of cognitive-behavioral therapy for depression and HIV medication adherence.

Stacey E. Prince, PhD, is in private practice in Seattle, where she works with individuals, couples, and groups, and specializes in the treatment of mood and anxiety disorders, recovery from trauma, relationship issues, and psychotherapy with lesbian, gay, and bisexual clients. She is also Clinical Instructor at the University of Washington, where she supervises clinical psychology graduate students. In addition, Dr. Prince is active in the Washington State Psychological Association and recently served as cochair of the Committee on Gay, Lesbian, Bisexual and Transgender Concerns. She has been involved in several National Institute of Mental Health-funded studies, and has published articles and book chapters on gender issues in depression, cognitive-behavioral therapy for depression, and integrative behavioral couple therapy.

Foreword

If there is a theme that characterizes the lives of lesbian, gay, and bisexual (LGB) individuals over the years, it has been that of invisibility. Because of the long and regrettable history of societal oppression of sexual minorities, a very clear message had been sent out: It is hazardous to your physical and psychological health to be anything but heterosexual. As a means of self-protection, individuals in the LGB community have traditionally found it necessary to hide this aspect of their lives.

Until recently, this theme of invisibility has also characterized LGB mental health professionals. Even at the risk of possibly marginalizing themselves professionally, an increasing number of LGB psychologists, psychiatrists, and social workers have now become more open in talking and writing about sexual minority issues. Indeed, it was largely through their efforts that homosexuality was finally removed as a DSM-diagnosable disorder. Although an extensive psychological literature on LGB issues now exists, this information has nonetheless remained invisible to mainstream psychology. LGB professionals have been telling what it is like to be part of a sexual minority, but mainstream psychology has not been listening.

Nowhere is this more a problem than in the field of psychotherapy. Because LGB individuals need to deal with the stressors associated with being a sexual minority, in addition to those life struggles confronting all humans, they are more likely to make use of psychological services. Unfortunately, the LGB community has not always received the best treatment from therapists. Quite the contrary, past surveys have shown that a number of LGB clients have been damaged by their therapeutic experiences. Even in more recent years, when therapists have developed a more positive attitude toward LGB individuals, the stance "I treat LGB clients the same way I treat my heterosexual clients" leaves something to be desired. The fact that therapists may be biased or unaware of the key issues confronting their LGB clients clearly reflects a shortcoming in the profession.

This book by Christopher Martell, Steven Safren, and Stacey Prince represents an important step in closing this gap between the mainstream and LGB literature. There exist cognitive-behavioral therapists who are quite knowledgeable about cognitive and behavioral interventions but know little about LGB issues. Other therapists are well aware of the challenges associated with being LGB but know little about cognitive-behavioral interventions. This volume serves the very important function of integrating these two therapeutic communities.

The lives of LGB individuals have improved over the past decade. Still, as a group, they continue to experience numerous psychological problems, the majority of which stem from those of us who are heterosexual. It has been estimated that one out of three gay youth attempt suicide, often as the result of family problems associated with their sexual orientation. One out of three gay youth are verbally abused by a family member, and one out of ten are the victims of physical abuse at home. Within the school setting, one out of four are victimized physically. That the aftermath of such experiences can take the form of posttraumatic stress, anxiety, depression, and substance abuse should come as little surprise. All this makes the need for this book that much more relevant, especially because cognitive-behavioral therapy has developed therapeutic methods for dealing with such problems.

Although informing therapists about the unique issues that confront LGB people is very definitely a step forward, more is clearly needed. The oppression and discrimination confronting LGB people clearly call for societal changes, without which even the best of our therapeutic interventions may be limited. Complementing the many LGB advocacy groups currently addressing this problem, a group of psychologists with LGB family members has recently been formed. The mission of AFFIRM: Psychologists Affirming Their Gay, Lesbian, and Bisexual Family (*www.sunysb.edu/affirm*) is not only to provide open support for LGB relatives but also to support clinical and research work on LGB issues and inform mainstream psychology about what is known about such issues. It is within this context that I am honored to offer this foreword to a book that serves this goal.

MARVIN R. GOLDFRIED, PhD
State University of New York at Stony Brook

Preface

Following the breakup of his 6-year relationship with his partner, Alex, Danny went through a long period of deep despair. Fortunately, a good friend of his had read about cognitive-behavioral therapy on the Internet and helped Danny find a well-respected cognitive-behavioral therapist who promptly set up an appointment. The therapist, a distinguished gentleman, was warm and welcoming. Danny told him about his breakup with Alex, and the subsequent sadness he had felt during the past 7 months. Danny was pleased with the therapist's calm demeanor, appreciating how he gently placed a box of tissues closer to his chair when Danny started to tear up. The therapist stated, "It sounds like you really loved Alex, and are grieving her loss. I do think you made the right choice to come to me because I think this is more than just grief. You are showing signs of clinical depression. The two of you were together for 6 years, and that is a long time, but whether you and she had been together for 6 years or 6 months, you are really struggling now that the relationship is over, and I think I can help." Danny was dumbstruck. He truly had believed that the therapist could help. At that moment, however, Danny's hope was lost. He shifted in his seat, cleared his throat, and said, "I'm sorry, I guess I didn't make it clear that Alex is a man, and he broke up with me because he fell in love with Ed." The therapist begged Danny's pardon and continued with the interview, somewhat sheepishly. Danny left the office and did not return for a second session.

THE REASON FOR THIS BOOK

Three contemporary assumptions provided the impetus for writing this book. These assumptions have not been articulated in professional journals or books, however. One either hears them anecdotally at conferences, or can infer them from reading books on lesbian, gay, and bisexual (LGB)[1] issues or training manuals in behavior therapy written as late as the early 1990s. Therapists trained in other approaches frequently make the first assumption: that cognitive-behavioral therapy (CBT) is a simplistic approach that does not take into account the complexity of human emotional experience. These therapists conclude that CBT cannot account for the complex experience of developing a sexual identity or becoming comfortable with one's sexual orientation.

Most of the literature on LGB issues is written from the perspective of developmental or social psychology. Furthermore, therapists working with this population have gravitated toward methods of treatment that are client centered. These trends lead many to the second assumption: that CBT has little to offer the LGB community. Only recently has a literature emerged that demonstrates the application of CBT with this population. For many young LGB therapists who have been trained as cognitive-behavioral therapists, it is difficult to find adequate supervision to work with an LGB population. LGB supervisors may introduce them to feminist theory and client-centered or other approaches but may be uninformed about CBT, leaving the trainee to grapple on his or her own to become competent in conducting CBT with LGB clients.

The third assumption, made by a small minority of theorists and practitioners, is that heterosexuality is the only mature sexual orientation and that LGB individuals are impaired in some way. Those who make this assumption either practice forms of therapy that attempt to change sexual behavior to fit a heterosexual stereotype, or, preferably, decide not to work with LGB clients.

The assumptions that CBT is a simplistic model, that CBT has little to offer the LGB community, and that LGB individuals are in some way impaired are currently present in professional circles. None of these assumptions, however, are accurate. It was the need to dispel these assumptions that motivated us to write this book. In doing so, we hope this book offers treatments that can help to improve the lives of LGB individuals.

The political climate changes frequently and differs from place to place. Same-sex marriage is now legal in Canada, a first in North America. Belgium and the Netherlands also recognize same-sex marriage. In the United States, however, the Defense of Marriage Act bans same-sex couples from enjoying most of the rights of married heterosexual people. And in some parts of the world, sex between people of the same sex is punishable by death. There can be great joy for LGB individuals who find freedom and love in their lives, but there can also be great sadness for those who are rejected by loved ones or who live in fear and anonymity. Contexts shift, and CBT is a treatment that can focus on the environmental and individual factors influencing each client. It is ideally suited for people who come from diverse backgrounds but share one bond in common: the desire to love in the way that feels natural to them.

Combining Literatures to Propose LGB-Affirmative Cognitive-Behavioral Therapy

There are many excellent books written on CBT for a variety of human problems. We have brought together this literature with the literature on LGB issues to present a CBT approach to the specific problems faced by LGB clients. Much of the literature on LGB adults has focused on understanding identity development, couple interactions, and the impact of stigma and oppression. Sexual minorities suffer from stress related to their sexual orientations, which may place them at increased risk for physical or mental health problems, in particular, depression and anxiety disorders (see Cochran & Mays, 2000; Cochran, Sullivan, & Mays, 2003; Gilman et al., 2001). LGB individuals frequently present with these problems in mental health clinics (e.g., Rogers, Emanuel, & Bradford, 2003). CBT can successfully treat a variety of such disorders, including substance abuse (Marlatt, 1985), anxiety disorders (Barlow, 1988), borderline personality disorder (Linehan, 1993a), chronic pain (Philips, 1988), couple problems (Jacobson & Christensen, 1996b; Jacobson & Margolin, 1979), depression (Beck, Rush, Shaw, & Emery, 1979; Martell, Addis, & Jacobson, 2001; Persons, Davidson, & Tompkins, 2001), insomnia (Morin, 1988), and obsessive–compulsive disorder (Foa & Kozak, 1986). Despite the success of CBT with these problems, there are few clinicians with expertise in both LGB-affirmative psychotherapy and CBT. Training programs that tend to focus on LGB-affirmative psychotherapy largely do not have adequate course work in CBT, and most training programs that focus on CBT do not have adequate course work in LGB issues (Anhalt, Morris, Scottie, & Cohen, 2003).

Recent approaches to the application of CBT interventions to sexual minorities are similar to applications of such interventions to individuals from ethnic or cultural minorities (Purcell, Campos, & Perilla, 1996; Safren, Hollander, Hart, & Heimberg, 2001). Just as therapies do not attempt to change one's ethnicity, cultural beliefs, or personality, CBT's purpose with sexual minority clients is to enhance psychological and behavioral functioning, rather than to change their sexual orientations.

Practitioners and proponents of behavior therapy and cognitive therapy have a long history of basing treatments on empirical findings.

Basic research on human learning as well as clinical research on psychotherapeutic outcomes has informed the development of the theories and therapies. Functional analyses, the hallmark of cognitive and behavioral therapies, take into consideration both the environmental antecedents to and the consequences of behavior. This emphasis on both the environment and the individual allows the cognitive-behavioral therapist to formulate a case conceptualization (Persons, 1989; Turkat, 1985). Traditional diagnosis of the client, environmental variables that have an impact on the individual, particular beliefs and attributes that may cause difficulty for the individual, and the behavioral repertoire available to the client all play a role in case conceptualization. A thorough functional analysis provides a basis for extending empirically supported protocols to individuals.

Clinical behavior therapy (Goldfried & Davison, 1976/1994) as a broad treatment approach utilizes techniques drawn from theories of reinforcement and social learning to treat a variety of disorders. In the late 1960s and especially in the 1980s, cognitive approaches that focused on the effects of thinking on emotions and behavior (Beck, 1976; Ellis, 1962) gained popularity among behaviorally trained practitioners and researchers. Today, behavior therapy and cognitive therapy are frequently recognized as complementary approaches, and are referred to as cognitive-behavioral therapy. CBT has great relevance to the mental health needs of LGB individuals. Not only is it effective in treating general psychiatric disorders and relationship distress, but it also provides opportunities for clients to learn coping strategies to deal with unique problems that stem from the stress of sexual minority status.

DEFINITION OF TERMS

The language used in discussing LGB issues can become cumbersome, complex, and individualized. We wish to clarify the use of terms and the constructs that are emerging from the current literature, as we attempt to follow culturally sensitive terminology. However, we wish to convey the understanding that many individuals who represent a sexual minority do not label themselves in the way that heterosexual society might label them. For example, in the HIV-prevention literature the term "MSM" or "men who have sex with men" has been employed to describe a *behavior* so that individuals who do not identify as "gay" or "bisexual," but who have sex with men, can still fit into a category that is understandable. Many African American men who have sex with men do not identify as gay, but use the term "on the down-low" as a way to refer to their behavior. Some men who have sex with other men, or would like to, furthermore reject being called gay or bisexual because they feel it implies that this is the central aspect of their personality. Similarly, women from some ethnic groups reject the term "lesbian" because it is seen as representative of the white culture, because they have no such word in their native language, or because cultural taboos about sexuality render them invisible within their ethnic group (Greene, 1994). Many young people who have same-sex sexual attractions are reluctant to place a label on their sexuality. For example, interviews with young women between the ages of 18 and 25 years with same-sex attractions revealed a range of responses to the question "How do you now identify?," with many participants disliking typically used labels like "lesbian" and "bisexual" (Savin-Williams, personal communication, 1998).

The term "homosexual" has come to be associated with pathology and is typically considered one of the least desirable terms to be associated with these populations. The American Psychological Association suggested that authors use the terms "lesbians, gay men, and bisexual women and men" to reduce bias in language in published works (American Psychological Association, 2001). However, using these terms implies that one is referring to a specific, homogeneous group. There are varieties of experience and multiple communities among those who identify as lesbian, gay, or bisexual. When we refer to the *LGB community*, we are referring to these many communities. There are also many different ethnic, racial, and cultural groups who must be considered in this discussion. Culturally, not all people who have same-sex sexual attractions or engage in same-sex sexual behavior consider themselves lesbian, gay, or bisexual. Although we use the terms "lesbian," "gay," and "bisexual"—and even shorten the term to the abbreviation (LGB)—it is important to note that this is a convenience for the purpose of writing, not the expression of a uniform reality for these diverse people.

The terminologies of *sexual orientation, sexual preference, sexual behavior*, and *sexual identity* are also often confused. The term "sexual orientation" refers to the direction of an individual's sexual longings and/or fantasies and attraction toward a male or female partner (Bell & Weinberg, 1978), usually an enduring and cross-situational experience (Martell, 1999). Sexual orientation may be enduring for some but not others, and there are many who believe that sexual orientation is more fluid along a continuum from exclusively lesbian/gay to exclusively heterosexual than it is static (Brown, 1995). "Sexual preference" is a term that has often been used interchangeably with sexual orientation, but the former is not a precise term because of the implication of choice, which has led to much misunderstanding of LGB people. The word "preference" suggests a casual liking or disliking of a particular activity or object, such as when one prefers to play racquetball rather than croquet, or when one prefers chocolate to lemon. "Sexual identity" is considered distinct from sexual orientation. Sexual identity has to do with self-recognition of one's sexual orientation and sexual behaviors and the meanings one places on them (Savin-Williams, 1990). "Sexual behavior" is self-explanatory and includes the sexual activities that an individual engages in regardless of the gender of the sexual partner. As we have stated earlier, a person's sexual behavior does not always coincide with his or her sexual orientation or sexual identity. For example, a man whose sexual attraction is primarily to women may engage in sex with a male partner because he enjoys certain pleasures this partner provides, but still identify himself as heterosexual.

Although much of this book addresses the individual differences among people who engage in same-sex sexual activity, we also refer to a particular, albeit broad, class of people when we speak of treatment. The various applications of CBT techniques with LGB individuals are discussed with the following assumptions about this population:

1. Individuals are gay, lesbian, or bisexual inasmuch as they identify themselves as such, either privately or publicly. Clinicians are cautioned, however, to recognize that not all individuals from all cultures will accept terms like gay, lesbian, or bisexual. In some Latino cultures a man may have sex with men but not consider himself to be homosexual if he is the active rather than the passive partner sexually (Zamora-Hernandez & Patterson, 1996). Likewise, the terms heterosexual, homosexual, and derivatives of these words that classify people in linear terms (either this or that) are not recognized in all cultures (Tafoya & Wirth, 1996). When working with people of non-European descent, clinicians should not assume that a person is uncomfortable with his or her sexual identity or behavior simply because he or she does not use the terms that are understood by the majority mental health community. Furthermore, clinicians must recognize that many clients have multiple identities (Tafoya & Wirth, 1996).

2. Some gay, lesbian, or bisexual persons do not identify as such because they are afraid to do so for a number of reasons. A young man may recognize a strong sexual attraction to other men, perhaps exclusively to men, but still not refer to himself as gay. Nevertheless, because he experiences these desires and feelings and may invest energy into either denying or hiding these feelings, he would still fit the definition

of a gay man. We would say this man is "in the closet," to use a popular expression.

3. Although one aspect of an LGB identity is to be part of a community of LGB people, we consider someone to be lesbian, gay, or bisexual regardless of his or her level of commitment to a particular community. Therefore, one could consider oneself to be lesbian, and be involved in women's groups and various activities, but have no allegiance to a particular lesbian community. Such a woman might attend a pro-choice rally, but would never march in a gay pride parade or socialize at lesbian bars. She may even have a primary relationship with a woman, but they may enjoy the friendship of mostly heterosexual people.

In sum, it is clear from this brief review that the concepts of sexual identity and orientation are extremely complex and that people do not fit into neat, distinct, categories. Throughout the book, we have tried to use terms consistently, although they may not reflect the experience of all clients who seek therapy. Clinicians need to ask clients about their individual experiences and to talk about their clients' sexuality accordingly, without making assumptions based on broad classes of sexual orientation.

STRUCTURE OF THE BOOK

Chapter 1 provides a general understanding of the unique developmental challenges faced by LGB individuals for readers who may be familiar with CBT but unfamiliar with LGB mental health. Chapters 2 and 3 then focus on behavioral assessment and basics of CBT for readers who may be familiar with LGB mental health but unfamiliar with CBT. We next focus on two highly prevalent sets of problems that respond particularly well to CBT: depression (Chapter 4) and anxiety disorders (Chapter 5). Because same-gender couples face challenges that mixed-gender couples do not, we have included a chapter on couple therapy (Chapter 6). Several other disorders commonly treated by CBT therapists, such as obsessive–compulsive disorder and posttraumatic stress disorder, are covered in Chapter 7. We also present issues raised by the HIV epidemic in the gay community and suggest ways in which CBT can help in both HIV prevention and HIV-related problems. Given that the fields of behavior therapy and CBT are dynamic, and new treatments and understanding of human behavior continue to evolve, we present in Chapter 8 some of the emerging trends in CBT. Chapter 9 addresses ethical principles in working with a LGB population. Finally,

Chapter 10 provides a brief overview of the past and a look ahead to the future of CBT with LGB individuals.

No single volume can provide all of the information necessary for conducting CBT with LGB people. It is our hope, however, that students, therapists, and researchers will find the empirically supported and clinically relevant, practical information in this book useful for treating their LGB clients.

Acknowledgments

My dedication to empirically based practice was influenced many years ago by faculty at Hofstra University, particularly Junko Tanaka-Matsumi, Mitchell Schare, Richard O'Brien, Robert Motta, and Howard Kassinove. I think I have emulated Andrew Berger, my role model for being an overworked psychologist, quite satisfactorily, and I am grateful for Andy's guidance in my early clinical training. Several people since then have helped me to develop my understanding of work with lesbian, gay, and bisexual adults, especially Laura Brown and Douglas Haldeman. The opportunity to write was first provided to me through my association with the late Neil S. Jacobson at the University of Washington. I am forever in his debt. My office partners at Associates in Behavioral Health in Seattle, Kim Collier, Thomas Land, Howard Leonard, Timothy Popanz, Stacey Prince, and Chet Robachinski, have shown constant patience with my preoccupation with writing and saying "yes" to time-consuming projects.

The Guilford Press has been a remarkable publisher. I've learned to appreciate the importance of a good editor. Jim Nageotte provided exceptional editorial advice from the inception of this work. The copy editor, Jacquelyn Coggin, the production editor, Anna Nelson, and the staff at Guilford all deserve our gratitude.

As the reader will see, behavior therapy is not static. Understanding evolves and new approaches to treatment are developed and evaluated. Several innovators and experts were kind enough to assist us with comments on our attempts to illustrate this with discussion of new treatments. I would like to thank Steve Hayes at the University of

Nevada, Reno, and Robert Kohlenberg and Amy Wagner at the University of Washington, for taking time to read short sections of the book and provide comments and suggestions. Kevin Kuehlwein at the University of Pennsylvania provided substantial comments on the first draft of the book that helped to clarify the final product.

My coauthors, Steven Safren and Stacey Prince, provided me with an ideal team with which to work on this project. Finally, my partner, Mark Williams, has been supportive throughout this process, accepting this book as a third party in the early years of our relationship. Partners, family, and friends tolerate our absences, distractions, and commitments apart from them when we engage in endeavors such as this. They, most of all, deserve our thanks.

—C. R. M.

I owe a tremendous amount of thanks to my academic mentors for their ongoing efforts in training and their collaboration throughout my professional development. Rick Heimberg, my graduate school mentor, allowed me to be part of his research program in the middle of my graduate school training, which afforded me the opportunity to learn and participate in an active clinical research program, while also supporting my own independent research and clinical interests. He continues to be a huge support to me in all professional areas. At Massachusetts General Hospital, Dr. Michael Otto is also a superb colleague and mentor, and I can't really imagine a better person to work with. I am also thankful to Jonathan Worth for all the support he has given me. Dr. Kenneth Mayer is probably the most productive researcher I know, and I (and the LGB community) owe him a great deal of thanks for his work in the area of HIV and gay men's health. I value his input, guidance, and of course, the opportunities that he has given me in my work with him at Fenway Community Health.

Finally, I also owe thanks to my life partner, Bill, for his continued support on this project (and on everything else), his tolerance, and his dedication.

—S. A. S.

I am fortunate to have had many outstanding clinical supervisors, research advisors, and mentors who shaped my professional development, in particular the late Neil Jacobson who was my graduate school advisor until his untimely passing in 1999. I would especially like to thank John Gottman and Andy Christensen for their continued support and guidance as I completed my degree after Neil's death; Judith Gordon, Pat Matthews, Christine Ho, and Pat Fallon for their outstanding clinical supervision from a variety of orientations; Corey Fagan for always supporting University of Washington graduate students in getting excellent clinical experience along with their research training; and Steve McCutcheon, who directs the outstanding Seattle Veterans Administration internship program.

Knowing that many of the problems faced by gay, lesbian, and bisexual youth and adults are due to lack of acceptance, I have felt so grateful for my parents' support from my coming out through my commitment ceremony. And, finally, I cannot express enough gratitude to my partner, Teri. Having lived through the rigors of my graduate training, she had been encouraging me to slow down and "just say no" to new projects, but in spite of that, has been unflinchingly supportive of this endeavor. Whatever I have learned through the research and practice of psychology, it's Teri who has taught me all the really important stuff about relationships.

—S. E. P.

Contents

COGNITIVE-BEHAVIORAL THERAPIES
WITH LESBIAN, GAY, AND BISEXUAL CLIENTS

Chapter 1

Specific Developmental Challenges for Lesbian, Gay, and Bisexual Individuals

To understand the nuances of problems with which LGB clients present, it is helpful to have a sense of the developmental hurdles and related identity issues these clients faced growing up. Ella's case illuminates some of these challenges. By the time Ella first sought therapy, she believed she had conquered many obstacles. Trying to play out her role in her aging parents' life, however, had proven to be more of an obstacle than the others. Now that both her father and mother required 24-hour nursing care, the burden had fallen on her to provide such services. She was glad to help them. Her parents had been mostly good to her, but Ella could remember a time when the relationship with her parents had been strained.

Ella was raised in a middle-class family. Her father was an engineer and her mother, a nurse. Ella had always felt different from her peers. Hers was the only African American family on her block, and she was one of only four African American children in her elementary school. An outgoing child, Ella made friends easily. When she talked about her childhood to her therapist, she said she had never been aware of racism in her school; she assumed it must have existed, but she had been oblivious to it.

When she started high school, Ella believed that race didn't matter. She just wanted to fit in with her peers. The student body at her new school included just 10 more students of color than in her elementary school. In high school, Ella had her first taste of racism when she began

1

dating. A good student and a strong athlete, Ella was proud to be captain of the girls' basketball team at her school. However, when she developed a crush on the captain of the football team, who was white, and he made it clear that he would never date her because she was black, Ella felt the difference between herself and her peers keenly. Her parents spent a great deal of time consoling her during this period. Her father related stories of how he had challenged racist practices in his profession in the past, and how he continued to face discrimination on his job. He knew he had been passed over for several promotions but never gave up, insisting on recognition for his abilities. After high school, Ella decided to attend a college with a high percentage of African American students, so she might feel she belonged. Her parents supported her decision, and Ella was accepted at a prestigious university.

In college, unfortunately, Ella's dream of belonging was not fulfilled. She had very little in common with many of the students who had grown up in larger urban areas. Eventually, she found a network of friends, mostly through her sports activities. During her junior year, she met Philip, a handsome, friendly, African American accounting major who was the star of the track team. They began dating and married a few months after both graduated. Both got good jobs out of college, which required a move to the West Coast. Again, Ella found herself in an environment in which she and Philip were in the minority, and most of her neighbors and colleagues at work were white. She felt like an outsider once again, but at least she had Philip on which to rely. She gave birth to their first daughter a year after they were married, and a son was born 2 years later.

Ella worked as a computer programmer and loved her work. She and Philip arranged their schedules so that they could have fewer child care needs. During her sixth year of marriage, Ella was assigned to a work team starting an exciting new project. The team leader was a very attractive woman named Sheila. Her beautiful gray-blue eyes and long auburn hair struck Ella the first time she saw Sheila. They were the only two women on the project, and they struck up an instant rapport.

When Sheila invited Ella out for drinks after work, Ella called Philip to make sure he could be home with the kids, then met Sheila at the bar she had suggested. She was so caught up in conversation with Sheila that she didn't even notice that there were no men in the bar. In fact, in recounting the story, Ella was embarrassed at how surprised she had been when Sheila told her she was a lesbian and was relieved that Ella was comfortable meeting her at a lesbian bar: "My eyes must have popped out of my head, I was so naive at that time. I'm surprised Sheila continued to speak to me at all after I had such a reaction." But the two did continue to speak. After a month on the project, Ella realized that she was falling in love with Sheila. She told her therapist, "It's not as if I'd never felt an attraction to a woman before. I always had at least one close girlfriend. But I had never fallen in love like that before. When I first started seeing Sheila in that way, I realized that I had not even been in love with Philip like that."

Within the year, Ella had come out to Philip, who, after initial surprise and disappointment, learned to respect Ella's courage in coming out and developed a strong friendship with her. Ella also told her parents about Sheila, but they were not supportive. They were happy to see Ella married, with two children. The last thing they expected was for her to tell them she was a lesbian and was leaving Philip for another woman. Her difficult years with her family began. Her brother, Germaine, would not allow Sheila to visit him. He and his wife had become very religious, and he told Ella that he didn't want his children to be "exposed" to her relationship with Sheila. Ella's children, however, were not concerned that their mother's new partner was a woman, and they enjoyed Sheila's company. They were still young when Ella and Philip separated, and Philip moved into an apartment only two blocks from Ella. It was important to them both that they remain close to the children. Ella remembered this period of her life, however, as one of great stress and sadness. She once again felt like an outsider in the mostly white lesbian community. She didn't like to identify as a lesbian. She had found it so difficult even to identify as an African American woman and to make meaningful social connections that the switch to this new community felt like a terrible challenge.

Ella's identity issues put a strain on her relationship with Sheila. They had tried to live together for a couple of years, but the relationship did not last. After their breakup, Ella dated several other women but was relatively content to be single. Philip had remarried and moved several miles away. Ella liked Philip's new wife, and they had very few conflicts over child rearing. Her children were now ages 14 and 12. Germaine and his wife and children had moved to the South. Ella's parents had, eventually, got used to the idea that she was lesbian and had even moved out West to be closer to her and the grandchildren. Because the health of both her parents began to fail at the same time, and somewhat prematurely, Ella felt the burden of needing to care for them. Germaine agreed to help out financially, but Ella was left to find proper care and a place for them to live. She felt that it was finally time to seek help from a therapist. Mainly, she believed she was going to fail her parents, and that she was an imposter, not competent to make the right choices. Ella was socially isolated and felt that she relied too much on Philip and his wife for emotional support. She told her therapist, "It has taken me 38 years to discover who I am, and I still don't really know where I fit in. I also know I can do my job, raise my kids, but at the same time, I feel like I'm ultimately going to screw up royally. I think these decisions about my folks are going to provide me with that opportunity to make a huge mistake that will result in something terrible. I really need someone to hear me and help me decide what to do."

Ella found a senior housing facility that provided a small apartment for her parents, with increased nursing care available. Her parents liked the location and were relieved that Ella lived within 10 miles of their new home. They did not discuss her relationships with women. Ella's therapist helped her to explore possibilities for becoming more connected with the LGB community, and Ella organized a book group with six other lesbian or bisexual women, two of whom were also women of color. Ella also spoke with her therapist about seeking a black church and speaking with the pastor about his or her views on LGB issues. She found a small church that was neither openly affirming nor hostile, but the pastor welcomed Ella and her children. She ultimately joined the choir and, through the church, enjoyed meeting new friends, who eventually tried to be matchmakers between Ella and other lesbian friends of theirs.

VIEWS ON DEVELOPMENT

Ella's story represents just one of myriad pathways to the development of a lesbian or gay sexual orientation. It also illustrates a debate about the development of sexual orientation and even the validity of using such a term at all. The debate involves two opposing perspectives: essentialism and social constructionism. The essentialist and constructionist viewpoints, from the perspective of providing cognitive-behavioral therapy (CBT), are important for therapists to understand for several reasons. First, simply taking a view that people will fall into a category of straight, gay, lesbian, or bisexual may preclude one from seeing individuals who do not define themselves in any of those ways, and could invalidate a client's experience. Second, a client's understanding of him- or herself is an important part of developing various beliefs about self and world that are crucial to cognitive and behavioral therapies. Third, cognitive-behavioral therapists who are not familiar with the literature on LGB identity should know that there is no agreement on how one should define sexual orientation. Some say it is fixed (the essentialist view); others say that all sexual orientation is socially constructed (constructivist view). Still others claim that it is fluid for some people and not for others.

The fundamental essentialist view is that sexual orientation is a more or less fixed state, and the property of one's sexuality resides within the individual person and is always there, whether expressed or not as heterosexual, homosexual, or bisexual. Genetic and environmental factors may play a part in the development of sexual orientation, but one's sexual orientation is determined by factors beyond the control of the individual and is a relatively stable characteristic. Ellis and Ames (1987) suggested that biological determination of sexual orientation takes place during prenatal development. Other essentialist views claim that inherited factors (Bailey & Pillard, 1991; Bailey, Pillard, Neale, & Agyei, 1993) have a role in the development of sexual orientations. The belief that variations in sexual orientation are cross-cultural and have occurred at different historical times and places, such as in Greece during the time of Plato, or in medieval Europe (Boswell, 1980), have been considered essentialist.

The social constructionist view rejects the notion that sexual orientation and identity are inherent in the individual, predetermined, fixed, or relevant for different cultures and historical epochs. Social constructionists reject notions of what they consider to be reified distinctions among heterosexuality, homosexuality, or bisexuality. In this view, none of these distinctions represents essential elements of human experience; they are instead socially constructed, as is the construct of gender (Kitzinger, 1995). To the social constructionist, it is impossible to talk of LGB individuals, because one cannot have a fundamental sexual nature that would lend itself to definition. Sexuality is therefore considered a social construction. They do not deny that there are varieties of sexual behaviors, but their view differs from essentialist interpretations of such behaviors. Ella's story provides an example of a woman who did not define herself in any particular way. Her sexual identity shifted as her affectional attraction shifted from Philip to Sheila. To the essentialist, Ella would be considered either bisexual or as one who recognized her lesbian orientation later in life. To the social constructionist, Ella's sexuality would be seen as fluid and not necessarily defined by any terms outside of her experience.

Resolution of this debate is, obviously, beyond the scope of this book; in fact, Kitzinger (1995) suggests that the debate is not resolvable. To most of our readers, the debate may seem more academic than pragmatic when it comes to working with clients who identify as LGB individuals. We define it here, however, because it is relevant to clients' understanding of themselves. Many, if not most, gay or bisexual male clients who so identify report experiencing sexual orientation as fixed. In discussing childhood history, these men report feeling attracted to members of the same sex since an early age. This, per se, does not imply essentialism. Some lesbian or bisexual women, however, report experiences different from those of men. Some women do not define their sexuality in terms of being straight, lesbian, or bisexual. They see their sexuality as determined by the person with whom they fall in love, not the sex of that person. Also, some women choose to be in relationships with women rather than men as a political choice, rejecting male dominance and oppression.

Garnets (2002) points out that the scientific community agrees that human behavior reflects both biological and environmental factors, and that there is no gene or prenatal hormone that controls human sexual orientation apart from the mutual influence of social and environmental factors. It is important to understand the complexity inherent in sexual orientation to grasp the multiple factors that influence development of a healthy sexual identity, whether the client is gay, lesbian, or bisexual, or chooses not to identify him- or herself by any such classification. Therefore, the CBT therapist cannot make assumptions about his or her clients' sexual behavior and orientation, regardless of the terminology clients use to describe themselves. It is important to understand each individual's experience, which makes the idiographic perspective of cognitive-behavioral assessment and treatment particularly useful.

No single theory of development can explain the multiple experiences of gay men, lesbians, and bisexual men and women. There is great diversity in ethnic and cultural variables, individual identity, and variations in communities in rural and urban settings. Some generalizations can be made, however, as a result of what has been learned about the developmental challenges of growing up as LGB individuals in a society that assumes that cross-gender sexual behavior and pairing is the norm. Depending on the culture in which one is raised, there may be more or less understanding of different sexual orientations. Almost all Western cultures assume that heterosexuality is the norm, and that children will grow up to pair with someone of the opposite sex. Although homosexuality and bisexuality are recognized and increasingly popularized in North America (e.g., in television shows such as *Ellen* or *Will and Grace*), it is extremely unusual for heterosexual parents to welcome and allow atypical gender behaviors or to encourage their children, if they suspect that the child may be gay or lesbian. Not all cultures share these sexual identities or make sexual distinctions in this fashion, however (Chan, 1995).

Some developmental models propose stages of coming in which people progress through a linear process: recognizing one's same-sex attraction, moving into disclosure and development of an LGB identity, then entering a unified LGB community. Many of these models, however, lack generalizable clinical and empirical support. First, they have largely been based on studies of white, middle-class males (Brown, 1995). Consequently, less is known about understanding sexual orientation differences between men and women, as well as for individuals of different ethnicity. Second, conflating individual identity development with group identity development confuses matters further in gaining a clearer understanding of this process (Fassinger & Miller, 1996). Third, the identity development literature has not included the experiences of people of color.

Using CBT with a mutually determined treatment plan and case conceptualization (instead of attempting to push someone through predefined stages) holds promise for LGB individuals, because it focuses on the individual case rather than relying on hypothetical group traits. From this perspective, the general understanding of LGB development can certainly inform a case conceptualization, but the specifics of each individual case must be examined carefully. Reynolds and Hanjorgiris (2000) warn that "in general therapists need to apply LGB developmental theories with caution. They need to evaluate whether the theory fits the client rather than try to make the client fit the model" (p. 50). Therapists need to be particularly sensitive to differences in cultural experiences regarding sexuality and sexual identity (Fukuyama & Ferguson, 2000).

SEXUAL IDENTITY IN YOUNG CHILDREN

Heterosexual parents have raised most LGB adults. In most cultures, distinctions are made between appropriate masculine and feminine behaviors, although the expected behaviors vary among cultural groups. Not all cultures see male and female as opposite ends of a pole, or as the only two genders. For example, many Native American groups accept individuals who are considered "two-spirited," possessing both male and female spirits (Tafoya, 1992). When children are raised in cultures that view masculinity and femininity based on biological sex, however, they are usually expected to fulfill the roles of their gender. Young boys are discouraged from playing with dolls, or wearing dresses or clothing considered "girls' clothes." To a lesser degree, young girls are discouraged from equivalent cross-gender behaviors. However, the term "tomboy," pertaining to little girls who enjoy the rough-and-tumble games usually reserved for boys, is much less pejorative than the corollary term "sissy." The more patriarchal the culture, the more embarrassing it is for a boy to act like a girl. When women and femininity are disparaged, boys or men who demonstrate cross-gender behaviors are also disparaged, and this may account for the fact that heterosexual men have more negative attitudes toward homosexuality than do heterosexual women (Kite & Whitley, 1998).

In the heterosexual household, the family typically assumes that all the offspring in the household will also be heterosexual. Family members and friends often tease little girls about whether they have a boyfriend, and boys about whether they have a girlfriend. Parents typically suggest future pairings with friends' children of the opposite sex, even with small infants. Although this is usually done in jest, the assumption is still clear. Little Ted will end up with little Mary, and he won't end up pairing with little Emilio. Heterosexuality is assumed.

For those young girls and boys who recognize differences in their preferences for cross-gender activities, or who are aware of same-gender attractions at young ages, the assumption of heterosexuality by their families can lead to great confusion. Few children think they will grow up to be LGB individuals. However, the child will become aware of appropriate gender behaviors, for example, that boys do not play with dolls, before they begin to recognize sexual attraction to specific individuals, male or female.

From a cognitive-behavioral perspective, the degree of punishment of cross-gender behaviors, or conversely, the amount of pressure to conform to gender stereotypes, by the family or other authority figures results in the child feeling more or less invalidated for his or her behaviors. Gay men and lesbian women often report having known that they were different from their peers at a young age (Gonsiorek & Rudolph, 1991). Without the pressure to conform to gender stereotypes or the expectation of heterosexuality, many of these children would have accepted their natural attractions as appropriate. When a boy is called a "sissy" or "faggot" and is told that it is unacceptable for him to play with dolls (perhaps with the exception of dolls that are marketed as "action figures"), he is punished for his behavior. Although he may stop the behavior, or take it underground by playing dress up only when alone in his room, the thoughts and feelings that seem natural to him will not go away; they, too, may simply go underground.

In many cases, as a result of this learning history, the child or adolescent begins to internalize the negative attitudes about his or her behavior. Developing negative attitudes about one's own LGB identity has been referred to as "internalized homophobia" (Malyon, 1982). In many cases, the term "phobia" would truly apply as the young LGB person works to avoid the appearance of being anything other than heterosexual. Shidlo (1994) suggests that internalized homophobia is associated with other psychological distress. Overt negative statements about other gay or lesbian people reinforce the child's secrecy about his or her own feelings. If, for example, a boy considered a "faggot" finds another boy who shows gender-atypical behaviors, then hurls similar insults at him, he is likely to be rewarded by his peer group of boys. Such behavior would also be negatively reinforced if the boy's anxiety over being the object of ridicule can be avoided by identifying himself as anti-gay. Similar phenomena can occur with girls as well.

Negative core beliefs about the self may develop along a paradigm that follows a pattern of increasing recognition of the self as bad or defective. First, a child recognizes him- or herself as different. Second, there is recognition that in social groups, being different is bad, and being "queer" is particularly bad. Third, the child recognizes that he or she is different because of same-sex attractions and/or atypical gender behaviors, internalizing the message "homosexual is bad," when the recognition that being queer is "bad" intersects with being different is "bad." The resulting belief that "I am bad because I am different and I am homosexual" can often be associated with a host of affective and behavioral difficulties, such as depression, social withdrawal, and avoidance of people associated with the gay or lesbian community (e.g., Meyer & Dean, 1998).

Many LGB children, unaware of their sexuality, nevertheless have a sense of themselves as being different from their peers. Early socialization shows children that being different is undesirable, and those identified as different are usually targeted for teasing or other abuse. Early awareness of being different can also bring an early belief that one is "bad." When a child grows to adolescence and does not completely fit with peers because he or she is not exclusively (or not at all) interested in the opposite sex, or in dresses or sports, or whatever the gender-appropriate behavior is for the particular social group, he or she may develop feelings of alienation and judge him- or herself negatively. Ongoing experience of being different can solidify beliefs of inadequacy or abnormality. The coming-out process may reduce the credibility of the belief that being an LGB individual is wrong as alternative beliefs gain increasing credibility. However, coming out does not always change the implicit beliefs that have been reinforced in the person's life, long before an awareness of sexual orientation. The belief that being different is bad can lead some openly LGB individuals to view themselves as impostors, carrying the tacit idea that they harbor a dark secret regardless of their being "out." The process of hiding one's true identity, even when it is in the person's best interest not to do so, reinforces a pattern of believing that should one be discovered, there will be negative social consequences. In some cases, this may be true, and it would not be in the person's best interest to disclose. However, when evidence points to the possibility that there will be support rather than censure, hiding may increase the individual's sense of being different, bad, or even a pariah.

It is important here to consider some basic facts about gender behavior. Behaviors observed in a young child are not necessarily predictive of future behaviors of the adult. Some young children who demonstrate gender-nonconforming behaviors will grow up to be gay or bisexual, and others will not. This is particularly true of girls: Gender nonconforming behavior in young girls is not predictive of adult behavior or sexual orientation. Additionally, many young girls and boys who demonstrate gender-conforming behavior do grow up to be LGB individuals.

Retrospective studies suggest a stronger correlation between adult sexual orientation and childhood gender nonconformity in men than in women (Bailey & Zucker, 1995; Peplau, Garnets, Spalding, Conley, & Veniegas, 1998). Gender nonconformity, furthermore, is not necessarily related to sexual orientation, and a man or woman may show great variation in gender behaviors but consider him- or herself to be heterosexual. There are also harsher biases against male gender nonconformity than against female nonconformity (Katz & Ksananak, 1994), which means LGB nonconforming boys are at greater risk of victimization than girls.

CLINICAL IMPLICATIONS OF SEXUAL ORIENTATION DEVELOPMENT FOR CHILDREN AND ADOLESCENTS

Understanding the complexities of growing up as LGB individuals will help therapists working with adolescents and adults. A CBT therapist will most likely be contacted by the parents of a troubled adolescent, or be sought out by an adult client. Knowing that an openly LGB adolescent or adult has encountered a variety of obstacles prior to making his or her way to therapy is important in developing the case conceptualization and treatment plan. Heterosexual authority figures may have reinforced negative beliefs about the LGB community; consequently, many young men first experience sexual contact with partners in furtive settings and/or anonymously. This has implications for these men's acceptance of their sexuality and is often in conflict with their ideas of moral behavior. There are also usually few options for LGB youth to begin to experiment with sex and dating in healthy ways compared to the many options provided to heterosexual youth. In summary, the therapist must consider the historical–developmental context of the client's behavior prior to making judgments about psychopathology.

COHORT DIFFERENCES IN SEXUAL
ORIENTATION DEVELOPMENT

Although generational differences are common among all groups of people, the differences are striking within LGB communities, because the political and cultural climate of tolerance and acceptance has changed radically over the last three decades. Men and women who came of age prior to the rebellion at the Stonewall Inn in New York's Greenwich Village neighborhood, in 1969, are now in their late 50s or older. These individuals grew up in a very different environment than that of the men and women who came of age after 1969, when the "gay rights movement" began, and social change allowed for open gay and lesbian lifestyles. The feminist movement also allowed greater flexibility in sex roles for people of either gender. Further change occurred when the first gay men were diagnosed with GRID (gay-related immune disorder), which later came to be known as acquired immune deficiency syndrome (AIDS) in the late 1970s and early 1980s.[1]

Now, a generation of young gay men has matured and come out in the shadow of AIDS. These gay men differ from their senior brothers, who are now in their 40s or older and survived the devastating loss of entire networks of friends and lovers. Younger gay men may either feel a sense of hopelessness and inevitability about AIDS or, alternatively, have unrealistic ideas about the effectiveness of the protease inhibitors to prevent AIDS-related disorders that have led to the death of so many. Although a variety of reasons beyond fatalistic attitudes increase vulnerability to behaviors that expose a person to human immunodeficiency virus (HIV), the practice of unsafe sex may be more casually accepted by younger gay men than by their older counterparts, who consider themselves to be survivors. However, when the sexual behavior of young gay men today is compared to that of their older counterparts when they were young, a reduction in high-risk sexual behavior is observed (Johnston et al., 1999).

Past research suggested that LGB youth may be at greater risk for certain psychological disorders, particularly suicidal ideation and suicide attempts. Although the data on lesbians are less clear, a study using a male–male twin registry of veterans who served in the U.S. military between 1965 and 1975 indicated that twins who identified as having had sex with another man at some point in their lives reported having had higher incidence of suicidal ideation or suicide attempts than their heterosexual brothers (Herrell et al., 1999).

Despite limitations of this study (such as the use of reported sexual behavior as indicative of sexual orientation, exclusion of women from the sample, and an ethnically homogeneous sample), the authors suggest that higher rates of suicidality are reported even when they account for the confounding effects of comorbid disorders such as depression and substance abuse. The higher rates of suicidality reported by Herrell et al. (1999) could not be explained by abuse of drugs or alcohol, nonsuicidal depressive symptoms, or other psychopathological diagnoses such as anxiety or personality disorders. Other studies have indicated that gay and lesbian youth are likely to report having attempted suicide more than non-gay counterparts (e.g., Remafedi, 1994). Social factors must be considered.

More recently, however, Savin-Williams (2001) has questioned the assumptions based on earlier data. He criticizes much of the published data on LGB youth suicide risk because of problems in sample selection, vague definitions of suicide, and use of unreliable measures of sexual orientation and suicide attempts. The samples in these studies are often drawn from settings in which self-identified LGB youth have sought support and help, such as crisis centers or runaway shelters. Savin-Williams conducted two studies to test his hypotheses about an overestimation of LGB individuals' suicide attempts. He concluded that by distinguishing false attempts from actual attempts and eliminating ideation alone from the definition of suicide, attempt rates were 13% for the young women in his study, which he states is only slightly higher than the rate reported for non-gay-identified youth. In a second study with both male and female participants, Savin-Williams found that young men who rated themselves a Kinsey 2 (predominantly heterosexual, but significantly homosexual)[2] were more likely to report a suicide attempt than other sexual minority male groups. Interestingly, Savin-Williams found that participants who identified themselves as gay or bisexual according to the Kinsey scale (Kinsey 3–6) were no more likely to attempt suicide than heterosexual participants (Kinsey 0). He concluded that professionals need to be aware that LGB youth in support groups may, in fact, be at higher risk of suicide, but that they do not represent all LGB youth, many of whom do not identify themselves as such. He also warns that self-identified LGB youth may be following a suicidal "script" developed from the oft-quoted data indicating that this group is at higher risk than heterosexual youth, thereby inflating their self-reporting.

Safren and Heimberg (1998) compared LGB youth in support programs to demographically similar youth in other types of support programs on suicidality and related variables. They found that there were zero-order differences between groups on depression, hopelessness, and suicidal ideation. However, when social support, coping, and stress were statistically controlled, these differences disappeared. This shows that other, environmental factors, and not sexual orientation, play a role in distress among this population.

Berman and Jobes (1992) identified eight risk factors in adolescent suicidal behavior: negative personal history, psychopathology, stress, behavior dysregulation, social/interpersonal isolation and alienation, self-deprecatory ideation, dysphoria, and hopelessness and method availability. Several factors that they identified are relevant for LGB youth, who are often socially isolated or alienated by their peers, particularly if they are open about their sexual orientation. Adolescence is a difficult time for most people. Problems often seem insurmountable. A young woman or man who does not believe she or he fits with peers may easily feel hopeless about her or his situation. Suicide could be seen as relief from a destiny of unhappiness. For many years, death by suicide or violence was depicted as the most common death for lesbian and gay characters in literature and film. Plays such as Lillian Hellman's *The Children's Hour* and Tennessee Williams's *A Streetcar Named Desire* (in which it is suggested that Blanche's "boy" killed himself after she saw him with another man and called him "disgusting") and *Suddenly Last Summer* (in which the gay character is cannibalized) are just a few examples. Gay men have often been depicted as lonely predators seeking young men or boys for sexual gratification. Lesbians are depicted as aging spinsters with little romance in life. In a study of homeless youth in Seattle, Cochran, Stewart, Ginzler, and Cauce (2002) found that LGB and transgender youth run away from home more frequently than their heterosexual counterparts and are victims of physical violence from family members (particularly for males) following a period of homelessness. LGB homeless youth also reported higher incidence of substance abuse, higher self-report ratings of symptoms of psychopathology, and more sexual partners than heterosexual homeless youth.

EFFECTS OF CHILDHOOD AND ADOLESCENT EXPERIENCES ON THE LGB ADULT

Whether future research confirms or challenges the notion that LGB youth are at higher risk for suicide, thankfully, the reality is that the majority of them will successfully grow out of adolescence and become adults. Many LGB adults also seek therapy at some time in their lives. Some data suggest that they do so at higher rates than heterosexual adults, which is particularly true for the lesbian community (Bradford, Ryan, & Rothblum, 1994; Cochran, Sullivan, & Mays, 2003; Jones & Gabriel, 1999). We propose three key reasons why LGB adults are seeking therapy at higher rates: (1) Their experience of being different has trained them to be more self-reflective; (2) they seek professional support because there is less natural support in their environment; or (3) they have greater distress in their lives.

Emerging research on the prevalence of mental disorders in LGB adults also points to the need to develop and adapt validated mental health interventions to the needs of these particular individuals. Gilman et al. (2001) recently analyzed data from the National Comorbidity Study and compared rates of mental disorders among people who have had same-sex sexual partners to rates among those who report exclusively opposite-sex partners. These data revealed higher rates of mood and anxiety disorders among respondents who had one or more same-sex sexual partners than among those who did not. One major limitation of this study, however, is that sexual orientation was defined exclusively by sexual behavior. Sexual identity was not considered, and there was no way for the authors to know whether identification as LGB individuals served as a risk or a protective factor. Another limitation was the small number of respondents reporting same-sex partners. Cochran and Mays (2000) also reported higher rates of depression and panic among men with same-sex partners, and higher rates of alcohol and drug dependence among women with same-sex partners. Cochran et al. (2003) found that gay and bisexual men were more likely than heterosexual men to be diagnosed with a mental disorder. Specifically, gay and bisexual men were 3.0 times more likely to be diagnosed with major depressive disorder and 4.7 times more likely to be diagnosed with panic disorder. Lesbian and bisexual women were more likely to be diagnosed with generalized anxiety disorder than heterosexual women. It is noteworthy, however, that approximately 58% of LGB participants in their sample did not evidence any of the five disorders assessed by the MacArthur Foundation National Survey of Midlife Development in the United States (MIDUS) questionnaire.[3] Although LGB individuals may be more vulnerable to behavioral health problems, a significant proportion of them show resilience and do not meet criteria for mental disorders.

Because CBT shows particular utility in the treatment of depression and anxiety disorders, these data point to the importance of assisting clinicians in the use of CBT with LGB individuals. Furthermore, the natural emphasis on the environment in CBT is important, because much of the difference between gay and non-gay populations may be due to environmental factors. Gilman et al. (2001) suggest several explanations for their findings: (1) Lesbian and gay men in general may have a higher incidence of psychiatric disorders as a result of the experience of discrimination, violence, and abuse, or low levels of social support; or (2) these individuals may simply lead riskier lives than their heterosexual counterparts.

Let's consider the first hypothesis, that lesbians and gay men have higher incidence of psychiatric disorders as a result of the experience of discrimination, violence and abuse, or low levels of social support. Despite changing societal attitudes toward LGB people that are making it easier for adults to live openly and express their sexual orientation, it is still difficult for LGB adolescents to cope with peer pressure and harassment. Whereas racial epithets are typically considered socially inappropriate in polite society, and children and youth in schools are openly discouraged from using them, or are punished for doing so, slurs regarding sexual orientation are common forms of verbal abuse among children and adolescents that seldom meet with adult attention or disapprobation. As a result, children or adolescents who are different or socially isolated in any way (i.e., not necessarily same-sex attracted) are frequently called "faggot," "fairy," "queer,"[4] or "dyke" as a means of insult and social control. When these insults are hurled at a young boy or girl who is beginning to recognize same-sex sexual desires, they can have greater psychological consequences. LGB youth typically maintain secrecy during their adolescent years. During a time when most adolescents are beginning to learn dating skills, and learn from important social and sexual bonds, LGB youth are frequently unable to do so fully because of the stigmatization involved in acknowledging their important homoerotic feelings. D'Augelli (1998) refers to "developmental opportunity loss" and "self-doubt induced by cultural heterosexism" as two results of victimization that LGB youth experience.

D'Augelli (1998) reported four types of victimization that can occur among LGB youth. The first, *marginalization*, occurs because these youths have fewer opportunities to explore their developing LGB identities without risk of rejection or violence by peers or families. The second form of victimization occurs when LGB youth experience *negative reactions from parents* and other family members about their sexual orientation, which can range from mild disapproval or refusal to discuss sexual orientation, to open hostility, physical violence, and/or banishment from the family. A third form of victimization is the *potential for HIV infection*, especially among gay or bisexual male youth. Practicing safer sexual behaviors, such as using condoms during anal and/or oral intercourse, requires negotiation on the part of both partners. The fourth form of victimization cited by D'Augelli is *direct attack*. He cites documented studies of assault on youth presumed to be LGB, on openly gay or lesbian college students, on young gay men in urban areas, and on young women. Comstock's (as cited in D'Augelli, 1998) analysis of victimization patterns among college students suggested that LGB students are victimized at four times the rate of the general college population. Many young LGB people are victimized by their families as well. Some are forced to leave home after disclosing their sexual orientation to their parents.

Whereas family, friends, and faith all typically provide means of solace, education, and support for most adolescents, many LGB youth are denied such support. They may have a restricted network of friends who are aware of their sexual orientation and guard their secret loyally. In rural communities, for example, it is common for LGB youth to believe that there are no other sexual minority peers in the community. In urban areas, there may be more support for openly LGB adolescents, but the risks of disclosure are still high. Youth may face particular challenges in families that belong to conservative religious groups, such as some Protestant Christian denominations (Hoge, 1996) or Orthodox Judaism (Dworkin, 1997), in which opposition to homosexuality is prevalent based on literal interpretations of scripture.

Whereas children and youth from other minority groups can rely on family to provide cohesion and support, LGB youth often hide their sexual identity from family or face rejection, if their identity is disclosed. It is important to note that youth of color face double or triple minority status (for lesbians of color) and have the added burden of self-identity that may be determined primarily by race/ethnicity, gender, or sexual orientation (Greene, 1994).

Therefore, it is probable that LGB clients will present in therapy with a history that includes some type of difficulty that they have either overcome or are struggling with as a result of being a member of an oppressed and often invisible group. There are also challenges that everyone typically faces at particular times of life. Among college-age LGB clients who may be considering career choices and finding a community of friends, as we noted earlier, some may be struggling with their sexual identities or trying to find a definition that they believe fits them appropriately.

The relevance of research on LGB adolescents and young people from a CBT perspective highlights how social learning, modeling, and other variables influence the development of negative core beliefs, or even conditioned emotional responses to their own sexual orientation. It is important to help LGB people find or create a life they value. CBT is ideally suited to this task. When clients struggle with reconciling their lived experience with the stereotypical ideas they have heard regarding LGB life, cognitive therapy can be useful in helping them evaluate their assumptions. Behavioral approaches can focus on teaching clients to accept their thoughts as thoughts, and not truths, and to act according to a value or goal (Hayes, Strosahl, & Wilson, 1999). When an LGB client finds it difficult to develop a social network, CBT can help him or her to decrease irrational and interfering fears, as well as learn prosocial skills and problem solving. Likewise, asserting oneself with family, friends, and employers is in the realm of behaviors that CBT therapists have seen and researchers have studied (see discussions on treating depression, anxiety, and couple problems; Chapters 4–6, respectively).

ISSUES IN LATER LIFE

There is much discussion of the aging "baby boom" generation (e.g., Roszak, 2001). Many "baby boomers" self-identify as LGB individuals, and many engage in same-sex practices without identifying themselves as such. These individuals face difficulties similar to those faced by their heterosexual counterparts. Like Ella, from the vignette at the beginning of this chapter, they must deal with elderly or infirm parents. Many have been involved in careers for years or have embarked on a second career. They may be trying to adjust to retirement. Many may have been in long-term relationships or in multiple shorter term ones. Some still hope to find love in their later years.

In citing research that suggests that gay men may believe they are beyond their prime earlier than their actual age would indicate, Barón and Cramer (2001) stress that clinicians must "be alert to the possibility that some clients may be prematurely aging themselves through beliefs" (p. 208). This phenomenon does not appear to be as common among lesbian women. Barón and Cramer suggest that aging LGB clients may be dealing with the issues of ageism, ableism (i.e., considering a healthy, physically able body as superior to one with disability or limitation), sexism, homophobia, and racism in some form.

It is important for the clinician to conduct a thorough assessment of the particular problems a client is experiencing. Clinicians must resist making assumptions about a particular client's experience simply because he or she identifies as LGB, or because he or she has sexual relations with members of the same sex. Reliance on overgeneralizations and stereotypes has led to many inappropriate and countertherapeutic practices with LGB clients (Garnets, Hancock, Cochran, Goodchilds, & Peplau, 1991). Proper assessment and case formulation are essential. To this end, we turn to the issue of behavioral assessment in the next chapter.

Chapter 2

Cognitive-Behavioral Assessment

Clinicians must conduct a thorough assessment prior to beginning any therapy. In this chapter, we discuss developing a case conceptualization (Persons, 1989; Turkat, 1985), components of cognitive-behavioral assessment, and clinical measures that are particularly useful with LGB individuals. By case conceptualization, we mean the individualized formulation developed by the therapist who has gained an adequate understanding of a client's problem list, as well as of environmental, historical, behavioral, cognitive, and physiological factors that play a role. Using this formulation to guide them, the client and therapist then collaboratively develop and agree on a treatment plan.

Most LGB clients present for therapy with problems similar to those with which their heterosexual counterparts present, and issues of sexual orientation are often secondary. Naive therapists can make the mistake of assuming that heterosexuality is the norm and therefore assume that whatever trouble the client experiences is because of his or her sexual orientation. On the other hand, therapists must take care not to ignore a client's psychopathology out of reluctance to recognize such in LGB clients (Gonsiorek, 1982). In this regard, when developing a case formulation, understanding LGB-affirmative approaches, while collaboratively developing a treatment plan that emphasizes treatment of the client's presenting problem, is key.

Heterosexual therapists often ask questions regarding sexual orientation development at conferences on LGB issues. One would therefore assume that their clients present with questions about how they became LGB individuals, or that most of these clients are questioning their sexual orientation; however, this is not likely to be the case. In fact, the 1991 survey conducted by the American Psychological Association's Committee on Lesbian and Gay Concerns identified several areas of bias in therapy, one of which was focusing on sexual orientation when it is not relevant (Garnets et al., 1991). However, when clients are questioning their sexual identity, or causal factors in their sexual orientation, CBT provides exceptionally useful techniques for helping them to resolve their questions and better understand themselves.

If LGB clients typically present with problems similar to those that heterosexual clients face, what does the therapist do differently in forming a case conceptualization? We suggest that the therapist use a culturally sensitive approach, similar to approaches employed with ethnically diverse clients (e.g., Fudge, 1996; Hatch, Friedman, & Paradis, 1996; Hayes & Toarmino, 1995; McNair, 1996; Tanaka-Matsumi, Seiden, & Lam, 1996). The preponderance of treatment techniques and assessment tools that assume heterosexuality makes it necessary to ensure that behavioral assessment is LGB-affirmative.

COGNITIVE, BEHAVIORAL, AND PHYSIOLOGICAL COMPONENTS OF PSYCHOLOGICAL PROBLEMS

We present several models of behavioral and cognitive-behavioral assessment, and their application to LGB adults. Various methods for conducting a cognitive-behavioral assessment exist. Practically speaking, the clinician cannot cover all of these areas with every client each time he or she conducts an evaluation and develops a case formulation. However, understanding the various processes that are of particular interest to behavioral and cognitive-behavioral therapists can inform the clinician trying to conduct an assessment for the first time. Broadly stated, cognitive-behavioral therapists look at three major components when evaluating patients for therapy.

Cognitive Component

Cognitive-behavioral assessment involves determining how individuals think in situations and what they believe about themselves, their world, their past, and their future. The cognitive component of psychological problems refers to the way an individual's thinking style and beliefs system play a role. Aaron Beck, the founder of cognitive therapy, delineates three levels of beliefs. Automatic thoughts are thoughts or images that are situation-specific—what is going through a person's head at the time he or she is distressed. Take the example of a socially anxious, gay man with low self-esteem in a bar setting. An automatic thought he might have on entering the bar would be "No one is going to like me." This level of cognition roughly corresponds to Freud's "preconscious," wherein thoughts are accessible but frequently just out of conscious awareness. The next level, underlying assumptions, has been defined as conditional beliefs, the rules by which one lives. Greenberger and Padesky (1995) suggest that underlying assumptions are usually stated in the form of "if . . . then. . . ." In a bar, a socially anxious, gay male interested in striking up a conversation with someone might think, "If I don't have a perfect opening, he won't like me," or "If I show anxiety, he will think I am weird." The third type of belief is a core belief, or schema, that is consistent over a number of situations and has a more absolute quality. The socially anxious, gay man in the social situation might have as a core belief, "I am inferior." In conducting a cognitive-behavioral assessment, the therapist should attempt to identify how an individual's thoughts and beliefs, and the resultant behaviors, serve to maintain his or her current problem. This would likely focus on automatic thoughts and underlying assumptions during the assessment and early treatment period, whereas core beliefs may not be identified until later, after seeing repeated themes across situations.

The Behavioral Component

The behavioral component refers to the way a person acts in a situation. For example, the socially anxious, gay man in a bar, given his beliefs about himself and others, and his thoughts in the current situation, may stand in the corner and avoid eye contact with others. As a result, people do not approach him. He therefore does not have the chance to obtain evidence against his negative beliefs or thoughts. In fact, after he leaves, he may interpret the fact that no one approached him as evidence that he is not an interesting or attractive person, instead of seeing the interaction as occurring within a system in which his own thoughts and behaviors have influence.

Physiological Component

CBT also considers physiological components of psychological problems as contributors to their maintenance. In depression, for example, physiological components such as fatigue, lethargy, and sleep problems can contribute to the maintenance of depression, in that they result in the person having low motivation to try to change his or her situation. In anxiety, such as that experienced by the gay man in the bar, physiological consequences such as elevated heart rate or sweating may cause him to feel even more anxious, because he believes that simply having or showing these symptoms constitutes a weakness.

THE ABCs OF BEHAVIORAL CONTROL

Behavioral therapy (vs. CBT) places a strong emphasis on antecedents, behaviors, and consequences, or the ABCs of behavioral control (Nelson & Hayes, 1981). It is in this area of assessment that most therapists inexperienced with LGB clients (regardless of theoretical orientation) make errors in diagnosis or treatment.

Antecedents

A behavioral therapist without training in LGB-affirmative therapy may see the client's current distress as a reaction to his or her sexual orientation. Although the research does not support such a conclusion, as we have noted previously, untrained therapists all too frequently focus on an LGB client's sexual orientation as the problem, or as the precursor to the problem (see Garnets et al., 1991). For example, the therapist may believe that the fact that a young man is gay is a direct antecedent to his difficulty in forming intimate relationships. The therapist's assumption that gay men are not capable of forming loving bonds with one another becomes confused with an actual antecedent to a problem behavior.

Behavioral analysis typically emphasizes current behavior and related antecedents (Hersen & Bellack, 1985). Although the client's history can inform the analysis, antecedents that are distal to the client's current complaint are highly subject to recall errors, lack clarity (Loftus, 1980), and are furthermore influenced by a person's life experience. Even in cases in which the event(s) occurred mostly as the client remembers, there is no way of knowing the intensity or frequency of the event(s) apart from the impact that remembering such events has on him or her. Therefore, during the assessment phase in behavioral analysis, the therapist refrains from making interpretations or suggestions, until a sufficient amount of information has been gathered.

The clinician can take into account the various life events reported by the client that have preceded development of a particular disorder. For example, if a client presents for therapy complaining of depression, the therapist will want to have clear descriptions of what the client means by "depression" and understand generally what the client's life was like prior to the onset of symptoms. Certain life events may have occurred that helped to instigate the depression. However, those events are not necessary precursors and cannot be used as complete explanations for the client's current presentation. Having said this, we also encourage clinicians to consider the impact of development on the LGB client, particularly as it relates to anti-homosexual bias in the culture in which most LGB people are raised.

Maintaining that sexual orientation must not be the focus of attention when looking for antecedents to client complaints is not to say that a client's sexual orientation is irrelevant. Here, we emphasize that one thing most LGB adults have in common is that people who identified as heterosexual raised them. This can result in their development in an invalidating atmosphere, which can result in negative attitudes toward oneself, isolation from peers, or psychological disorders such as depression and anxiety. Frequently, LGB clients, and particularly gay men, tell of a period in adolescence or early adulthood when they hoped that their attraction to people of the same sex was only a phase. To them, the period of "coming out" as gay or bisexual may have been a time of emotional turmoil (DiPlacido, 1998). This turmoil may be, although is not necessarily, a distal antecedent to distress. Depending on other environmental and internal factors, such as the reactions of others, the interpretation of these events, or the degree of invalidation perceived by the LGB individual developing in a predominately heterosexual environment, an individual could develop a cognitive vulnerability to depression. As a result of feeling different, he or she could take on negative core beliefs about him- or herself. Core beliefs are particular ways of seeing the self or the world that have developed early in life and are usually held as absolute (J. S. Beck, 1995). LGB individuals who develop in a society that assumes people who are not heterosexual are abnormal are vulnerable to developing negative core beliefs about being sinful, unlovable, defective, inevitably doomed to die of AIDS, or otherwise inadequate.

Most CBT interventions target specific behaviors, regardless of the diagnosis with which the client presents. Therefore, proximal antecedents are the focus of treatment. For example, a young woman may present to therapy with complaints that she has trouble with relationships, feels depressed most of the time, and has begun to stay at home and drink wine on weekend evenings. She may also tell the therapist that her earlier relationships with women, particularly her mother and older sister, were tumultuous. Regardless of whether further assessment leads to a diagnosis of major depression, dysthymia, substance abuse, an adjustment disorder, or even borderline personality disorder, the cognitive-behavioral therapist needs to determine the contexts in which behaviors that lead to problematic relationships occur. The therapist would therefore spend less time discussing with the client the possible distal variables, such as the bad relationship with her mother, unless she still has frequent, ongoing contact with her mother. Instead, the therapist would assess current relationships that are not satisfying to the client, and would specifically want to know whether there is objective evidence that this client has particular problems in relationships, or whether it is more a matter of the client's belief that relationships do not work out.

Behavior

The definition of "behavior" is not as simple as it may seem. Common-sense notions indicate that behavior is what can be observed, or that which is public. In CBT, emphasizing the cognitive, behavioral, and physiological aspects of psychological problems, "behavior" is defined as what the person does in response to certain situations. From the perspective of radical behavioral therapy, therefore, human behavior also includes verbal behaviors. Many of these behaviors are not public, but private; therefore, "cognitive" variables, to a radical behaviorist, are considered forms of behavior. Behaviorists refer to cognition or thinking as private behavior.

Although CBT in the broad sense has always considered both the public behaviors of an individual and the private cognitions, there has been disagreement over how to address properly the issue of private behaviors. Cognitive therapists have rightly understood that what people think often influences how they feel and act. The influence of cognition on behavior is not always a one-to-one correlation, however, as attitude researchers have argued for years (e.g., Bem, 1970). Behavior analysts argue that cognition cannot be seen as causal or antecedent to other behaviors, because it is itself a behavior. They argue, therefore, that a thought prior to a behavior is a behavior–behavior relationship, not an antecedent–behavior relationship (Hayes & Brownstein, 1986). So, to the behavior therapist, assessment of behavior includes both covert behaviors (thinking) and overt, observable behaviors.

Consequences

The consequences of a behavior are the events that follow it. Like the behaviors themselves, consequences can be public or private. Writing a letter about one's romantic feelings for a same-sex partner is public. Even if no one sees the writing or the letter, the act of writing it could have been observed. A woman feeling very frightened upon telling her parents about her attraction for other women, however, would be a private consequence. This consequence may lead to another public behavior, such as shaking or sweating, but the fear itself, or the thoughts accompanying the fear (e.g., "If I tell them, they will stop supporting me") are private consequence that are not observed by anyone other than the individual feeling the fear.

The consequences of a behavior either reinforce the behavior, increasing the likelihood of recurrence, or punish the behavior, decreasing the likelihood of recurrence. If, as a consequence of a behavior, something positive happens, then that behavior is positively reinforced. For example, assume that a woman's parents do not know she is attracted to another woman, and she is at home engaging in a conversation with her mother (antecedent). She tells her mother that she has recently begun to be attracted to a woman, and that she thinks she may be lesbian (behavior). Her mother responds favorably, saying that this is not what she would have chosen for her, but she respects her ability to understand herself and make good choices (consequence). Subsequently, the woman invites her father to dinner, with a plan to tell him about her sexual orientation and newfound love interest. In this case, the woman's behavior, telling her family, was positively reinforced, because it increased as a result of the addition of a pleasant consequence.

If, in this same situation, the woman feels more nervous about bringing up the issue now, because she learns that her mother is angry about her sister considering moving in with a boyfriend (a private consequence of the behavior of seeing her mother angry at her sister), the different context changes the antecedents that may lead to other behavior. If the woman quietly does the dishes (avoidance) and feels slightly relieved (a consequence of doing the dishes), we would say that the removal or decrease of her anxiety was a negative reinforcer. If she continues the behavior of doing the dishes in this interaction with her mother, we know that her behavior was reinforced. If, on the other hand, she told her mother, and her mother's response was hostile, accusing her of being perverted, and she subsequently decided not to tell her father or anyone else in her family, we would say that her behavior was punished. For some individuals, this entire process can happen without their ever physically entering the situation. If the woman *plans* to tell her mother about her attraction to another woman, for example, and *imagines* her mother being hostile and unsupportive, she may avoid telling her and continue to believe that she could not possibly let her family members know, because they are so hostile. She may continue to behave as though this were true, without ever checking it out with her parents.

In cognitive-behavioral assessment, these simple ABC patterns form the basis of understanding why clients do the particular things they do. However, as the example of the woman telling her parents about her sexual orientation illustrates, these patterns are more complex than they initially appear. The woman's mother responded in a hostile manner toward her, thus punishing (reducing the likelihood of recurrence) her attempt to speak openly with her mother. The complications in assessment arise in determining what actually happened versus what the client perceived to be happening. If, indeed, her mother stated that she was "perverted," we would say the simple ABC analysis is sufficient. However, if her mother was making a facial sneer for some arbitrary reason (clearing her throat, swallowing, squinting to see better in bad light, etc.) and the client only perceived this to be her mother's hostility, another important variable is added to the assessment. The learning history of the client will have conditioned certain responses on her part, as well as typical ways in which she perceives her environment. From the broadened perspective of cognitive-behavioral theory, the perceptions of the client fall under the category of organismic variables that also have to be considered in a behavioral assessment.

Cognitive therapy has suggested that one way to understand a client's learning history is to understand how he or she perceives him- or herself, the future, and the world. For the cognitive therapist, it is important to understand the antecedent events, the beliefs of the client, and the consequences of the belief. Ellis (1973) referred to this process as the ABCs[1] and stated that point A (what we have earlier referred to as antecedent) includes some "activity, action or agent that the individual becomes disturbed about" (p. 57). Ellis also refers to point A as the *activating events* that lead to a certain belief. *Beliefs* can either be rational or irrational. There may be an emotional or behavioral *consequence* of holding a particular belief.

People develop core beliefs or schemas that can lead to biases in the way they interpret information. Cognitive theorists consider these core beliefs to be cognitive structures or organizations that influence the gathering, processing, and recall of information. There are also stereotypical ways of processing information, such as self-referential thinking arising during times of psychological distress that influence interpretations of events. Finally, cognitive theorists look at cognitive products, such as the automatic thoughts and self-statements that an individual produces throughout the day (Blankstein & Segal, 2001). From a CBT perspective, a client may not always report the consequences of his or her behavior accurately, because the experience of consequences is itself subject to interpretation.

THE SORC MODEL

Goldfried and Sprafkin (as cited in Hersen & Bellack, 1981) have suggested that a thorough behavioral assessment must consist of an assessment of the stimulus, organism, response, and consequences. They proposed the acronym SORC as a reminder to the clinician to consider these four areas in assessment. SORC is similar to the ABC model described earlier. The *stimulus*, also called the antecedent, consists of the environmental variables that have an impact on a certain behavioral response. From a CBT perspective, behavior is situation-specific. People behave differently in different contexts; therefore, the clinician must be aware of the context in which the behavior is occurring. The *organism* is the person, and the clinician must understand elements of the individual's learning history that are unique. Person–environment transactions occur constantly. There are behavioral, cognitive, and physiological *responses* in this transaction. The clinician must understand the individual propensities of a particular client, as well as his or her beliefs and ideas about self and the world. Knowing what behaviors the client has engaged in historically can help to predict future behavior under similar stimulus conditions. The response is the target behavior, and *consequences* of the target behavior are the positive and negative outcomes that will either maintain or extinguish the response.

The SORC model can be directly applied to the experience of LGB individuals. There are many conflicting messages about LGB people in the media, in religious arenas, and in families. These messages can often be a multifaceted situation (S) that evokes a variety of responses from LGB people. A client may come to therapy with many self-defeating ideas about being gay, lesbian, or bisexual. It is, therefore, an essential part of evaluation to understand the "O" in the SORC model when working with this population. Therapists must also look at how the client responds to the situation, and his or her interpretation of the situation. For example, does he or she begin to withdraw socially, or to behave in an aggressive or hostile fashion? The consequences of the client's behavior will determine whether he or she maintains the behavior (if it is reinforced) or stops the behavior (if it is punished).

Thomas, a 41-year-old, gay, male client, provides an example of the importance of understanding learning history when doing a behavioral analysis. Thomas originally sought therapy because he had been feeling depressed. He and his partner were in couple therapy, and their therapist had suggested that Thomas seek therapy individually for his depression. The situational variables were as follows: Thomas worked as a manager in a company whose office building was badly damaged in an earthquake. The human resources department moved the executives to what the employees considered to be posh offices in a downtown building. However, they moved Thomas and his fellow managers to a large, windowless warehouse, with office cubicles set up. The company told these managers they would remain in this facility for at least 2 years, until reconstruction was completed on the original building. The summer months were coming on, and Thomas was looking forward to welcoming the sunlight after a long, gloomy winter. The prospect of spending 8–10 hours a day in a windowless building was upsetting him. Furthermore, he and his partner of 6 years were having relationship problems following his partner being laid off from work. After a long day in the new office space, which he referred to as "the warehouse," Thomas would come home, and his partner would reprimand him for not taking out the garbage or cleaning up the clothes in the bedroom. They had an argument about something nearly every evening.

Thomas told his individual therapist that he was feeling very sad and hopeless. This feeling state was the response component of the SORC model. He would try to ignore his partner and take a nap as soon as he arrived home. Thomas historically had never dealt with conflict. He stayed in his room whenever his parents argued. In high school, he accepted grades that he believed were unfair rather than discuss his concerns with his teachers. The consequence of this response was that his relationship with his partner deteriorated as emotional distance between them increased. Negative beliefs about a situation, and patterns of withdrawal and avoidance, can keep an individual stuck in a depressive cycle. Thomas also remained in his current job. Because of depression, and accompanying symptoms such as low motivation, he did not engage in problem solving to improve his situation; therefore, he did not get ideas for a solution to spending the next 2 years in a job that felt increasingly intolerable because of his reaction to the change in environment.

The organismic variables were similar to what clinicians hear frequently from depressed clients. The cognitive component (one of the relevant organismic variables in this case) may be illustrated as follows. Thomas interpreted being moved into the large warehouse as an indication that his company didn't appreciate his and other managers' hard work. He believed that he was seen as being expendable. He also thought his partner didn't understand how difficult it was to spend a day at this office, and he believed his partner would hound him less about chores if he really understood and cared.

Thomas's family history was likely a contributing factor to his vulnerability to becoming depressed under the current circumstances and illustrates how one's cognitive style can develop as a result of learning history. He had been raised in a religiously conservative family in which banishment from family events was a means of control. Thomas's parents frequently punished him: They would send him to his room to read the Bible and pray after minor rule infractions, such as not eating all of his vegetables or being slow to hang his coat in the closet. If he got poor grades in school, his parents would ground him for a week. To Thomas, both his employer's and his partner's behavior were similar stimuli for the response of retreating, as he had been trained to do as a young boy.

Thomas also shared his parents' religious convictions when he was a young man. He attended a religious college and had hoped to enter the ministry. His plans to enter the ministry changed when he had his first sexual encounter with a fellow male student and began accepting his sexuality. He had tried to ignore his sexuality prior to meeting this young man in college and, subsequently, felt terrible guilt about his sexual behavior. He believed that being gay was contradictory to the teachings of his church. Furthermore, he was convinced that violating the teachings of the church was tantamount to offending God, and destined him to a life of sin and unhappiness. He therefore ended the affair with the young man after a month. He tried dating a young woman during his senior year of college but was unable to become sexually aroused with her. They dated for 4 months, and the issue of sex was not discussed, because they both expressed the desire to refrain from sexual activity until after marriage. This conveniently allowed Thomas to avoid dealing with his sexuality for a few more months. Eventually, however, Thomas realized it would be devastating to this woman for whom he cared to pretend to be something he was not. He told her he was gay, and she suggested they could "work it out with God's help." He subsequently tried through prayer and "willpower" to modify his desires and orientation, but his failure to suppress his sexuality resulted in feelings of self-doubt and worthlessness, and eventually he came to realize that his sexual orientation could not be changed through prayer.

Thomas's parents were not as understanding as his ex-girlfriend. After college graduation, he decided to tell his parents about his sexuality and to move to a city where he could begin to understand this part of himself. His father wanted him to pay back all of the tuition money they had paid for his "wasted education," now that he was gay. His mother cried inconsolably for an entire evening. Both parents told Thomas they would pray for him and ask God to deliver him from this curse of Satan. Although his parents continued to express love and concern for Thomas in other ways, they never spoke of his sexuality again and would change the subject if he tried to talk with them about his dating life or current partner. (His parents' modeling avoidance of conflict is another important aspect of Thomas's learning history.)

Thomas had doubts about his religious upbringing and no longer attended church when he moved to the West Coast and openly acknowledged his sexuality. That was 12 years prior to the present therapy. However, the dramatic change in his job situation and the unhappiness at home triggered his core belief that he had lost favor with God as a result of his sexual orientation.[2] Thomas also believed that he was depressed because he no longer had a spiritual life. His guilt had begun to resurface, and his sexual life with his partner was compromised. He no longer initiated sex with his partner and refused any form of sex other than mutual masturbation, which he believed was "less dirty" than other forms of sex. His partner was very frustrated and criticized him for this behavior. In fact, his partner's ongoing sexual frustration and feelings of rejection may have correlated with his generally critical attitude toward Thomas. His partner's criticism of him felt similar to that of his parents. Thomas began to think that his problems were due to being inferior and had nagging doubts that his inferiority was due to being gay.

Thomas had both practiced avoidance and been trained to avoid by his parents. He had also developed many dysfunctional ideas about the religious significance of happy or unhappy life events. Now that he was unhappy with his workspace and there were difficulties with his partner, he interpreted these circumstances as indications that he would indeed have an unhappy life, and that this was the penalty for having tried to be gay. It is important to note that Thomas stated as much in therapy, and would also say, "I know this is ridiculous, but I still believe this to some extent." His ideas and behavior had been learned over many years and played a significant role in his response to current life events.

CASE FORMULATION

Behavioral assessment is an ongoing process, and the therapist will always revise his or her understanding of the client as new information emerges. When the therapist completes an initial assessment using one of the models discussed earlier, he or she can then begin to complete a case formulation (Persons, 1989; Turkat, 1985). In most cases, CBT therapists offer some part of the formulation to the client verbally or in written format for his or her feedback, then work in collaboration with the client to revise the formulation. A case formulation consists of several elements. Although behavior therapists originally emphasized diagnosis less than did other mental health practitioners, years of research into treatments for particular disorders and the need for diagnosis in third-party reimbursement have made traditional psychiatric diagnosis a standard part of any CBT formulation. However, CBT clients are not seen in terms of their disorders per se. Rather, they are seen as people with problems, and it is important that the clinician consider how this particular client experiences the disorder at this time. CBT therapists may, nevertheless, have rough formulations for many common disorders in terms of what behaviors, beliefs, emotions, history, and physiological symptoms are often found. In this way, therapists begin to watch for the types of issues that are likely to surface with individuals presenting with particular diagnoses, while not losing focus on the particular individual's idiosyncratic presentation.

The diagnosis, then, is only the first step in developing a case formulation that entails many hypotheses that must be spelled out in collaboration with the client over time. The second part of a case formulation is to develop targets for treatment, which may consist of behavioral changes that the client wishes to make, or that the clinician believes the client needs to make (but may not acknowledge initially). Irrational or maladaptive beliefs and attitudes may also be targets for treatment. In some cases, emotion regulation is the target. It is clear how the SORC can be very helpful in identifying treatment goals for therapy. Persons (1989; Persons & Davidson, 2001) also suggested that the clinician develop a problem list for each client to use as a means to guide treatment.

The Problem List

Cognitive-behavioral therapists are not as rigidly structured or clinically cold as the stereotype of them suggests, or as many believe. The development of a problem list is a good example of how the CBT therapist listens carefully to the client, extrapolates from what the client says, suggests treatment goals to the client, then plans particular interventions that are tested along the way for effectiveness. A therapist can develop a problem list by allowing the client simply to tell the story of what brings him or her to therapy, with a few directive questions to make sure that the therapist is clear on the particulars.

Alana sought the help of a therapist because she was told she needed to improve her attitude at work or risk losing her job. The following exchange demonstrates how the therapist listens for the problems to go on the list, then collaborates with the client to identify treatment goals.

THERAPIST: So can you tell me what has been going on recently that has led to your coming to see me?

ALANA: Well, as I told you over the phone, I'm basically here so I won't lose my job. My boss tells me I have to improve my attitude. I guess she's right. For the past year or more, I've just hated my job [a possible behavioral intervention to problem-solve the job situation]. I work in retail and have been making less and less money over time, because I just can't get into it [may indicate anhedonia and possible depression]. I have been selling clothes to teenage boys, basically, for 3 years. Isn't that ironic? I really couldn't care less what teenage boys wear.

THERAPIST: Have you tried to work in other departments?

ALANA: I don't see the point [suggests hopelessness], since I don't really care about any of it. I'm not a very good capitalist, and here I am in retail.

THERAPIST: How did you end up in that job?

ALANA: I was in college for about a year and wasn't doing very well. I got a little bit messed up over a girl; it was my first real relationship with another woman. Also, she and I were smoking a lot of pot at the time [indication of need to assess further substance abuse]. I couldn't get into school [possibly an indication of long-term dysthymia], so I quit after the first quarter of my second year. I needed a job, the store was hiring, and so I took it. That girl and I broke up, and I stayed on the job. I actually liked it at first. I thought I was selling some pretty cool stuff. The guys that come in are usually pretty cool, too. It just seems that as I've gotten older, they seem immature to me.

THERAPIST: Is there anyone special in your life now, or was the girl in college your last relationship?

ALANA: Oh, there is someone special. I have a partner, Lilly. She's great. We have lived together now for about 2 years. She's had a better job than I have; she works in computers. Times have been a little bit rough, though, because we had decided that we'd like to have a kid. Well, Lilly wanted one more than I did, and she wanted to get pregnant. She had been discussing coparenting with this gay friend of hers she's known since they were in high school. So she got pregnant but had a miscarriage about 2 months ago, after 5 months. It was pretty tough. [Alana's blue mood may be a result of grief over the loss of her partner's baby.]

THERAPIST: I'm very sorry; that does sound pretty tough. How have you and she been dealing with that?

ALANA: She's taken a leave of absence from work. That has made it hard, because we're pretty much relying on my salary, which is a lot less than hers. She cries a lot. I think she's depressed. So I guess when I go to work, I just can't get into it. I don't care about selling clothes when there are so many important things in life.

THERAPIST: Alana, it sounds to me like there are several things going on for you that may be helpful for us to work on [makes a "capsule summary" for Alana]. If I could list some of those things that I'm hearing as I listen to you, do you think it would be helpful?

ALANA: Sure, because I feel like I'm just rambling.

THERAPIST: Clients often feel that way, but I think you're telling me many significant things. It sounds like there may be several problems here. You are unhappy in your job, and perhaps it is time to talk about considering other options. Certainly, you've been feeling depressed and blue, and that has been going on for a very long time. It seems to have gotten worse lately as a result of your partner's miscarriage. I wonder if your bad attitude at work has been made worse by the loss of this baby.

ALANA: Well, it certainly didn't help anything.

THERAPIST: So those are several areas that I'd like to work on. You also said that in college, you and your girlfriend smoked a lot of pot, but what about now? Do you smoke pot much these days?

ALANA: No, not pot. Since Lilly lost the baby, though, I've been drinking more than usual. I get a little tipsy three or four times a week. It helps me to sleep, which has been difficult.

THERAPIST: Here are several more areas for us to discuss; perhaps you are drinking to escape from some bad feelings and need to learn to soothe yourself.

ALANA: If I could do that, I'd be much better off.

THERAPIST: It also sounds like sleep is a problem. So here we have about six areas to focus on. I would like to try to set some goals for our therapy in the next few sessions. Given what we've discussed today, what do you think might be good to work on first?

ALANA: I don't really know, but I just wish I could feel better.

THERAPIST: So maybe we can begin by talking about how to deal with your feelings in a healthier way than through using alcohol.

ALANA: That's as good a place to start as any.

The therapist can use this conversational style with a client to refine the diagnosis and to begin to formulate ideas for change. We discuss treatment strategies in later chapters, but the problem list can help to set the targets that determine the kind of interventions that can be tried with the client.

Arnold Lazarus (1971) proposed an acronym for assessing and treating clients. Lazarus's acronym, BASIC-ID, provides a comprehensive approach to assessment. The acronym stands for the following processes to be evaluated: behavior, affect, sensations, interpersonal relationships, cognition, imagery, and drugs. The word "drugs" is used as convenient shorthand for biological processes, completing an acronym that is more easily remembered. Although this useful acronym reminds clinicians to conduct a complete assessment, there is a great deal of overlap across these areas. For example, imagery is an important process to assess, especially when working with anxiety-disordered clients, but it is not necessarily distinct from cognition. Keeping in mind that clients may be troubled by particular images, memories, and interpersonal contexts, and that their biological functioning all has an impact on their presentation and the case formulation, helps the clinician to conduct a comprehensive evaluation and can inform the treatment plan.

FUNCTIONAL ANALYSIS

Our clients are complex; there is often more going on with them and their lives than meets the eye. A therapist needs to conduct a functional analysis of behavior and cannot always take a behavior at face value (Morganstern & Tevlin, 1981). In distinguishing the function of a behavior, however, the clinician must take care not to become overly deductive and make the error of seeing an underlying issue in every overt behavior. For example, a young man with an elevator phobia may simply be afraid of elevators, and his avoidance of elevators may simply function to keep him safe from the feared circumstance. However, another individual's avoidance of elevators can serve a completely different function. For example, when this young man avoids getting an advanced job in the finance industry out of fear of the job but states this fear as an inability to work in a tall building, where he would be forced to take an elevator, the function of the elevator fear is to keep him out of a scary job. Similarly, therapists frequently hear gay or lesbian people say that they are not "into the scene." The therapist can then assume that the client simply does not like to go out to gay or lesbian clubs. However, a good functional analysis of the behavior is necessary to understand this behavior fully, and it may reveal other functions. Consider the following exchange:

CLIENT: I have other lesbian friends, but I'm just not into the scene and don't go out much. I don't know where I'd meet someone to date.

THERAPIST: When you say you're "not into the scene," what does that mean?

CLIENT: Well, I don't like to do the big political lesbian thing. I'm not about to march in the pride parade, and I don't even like to just go to lesbian bars.

THERAPIST: Do you like to go to straight bars?

CLIENT: No, I don't really like to go to bars at all.

THERAPIST: So, when you tell me this, I wonder if you don't like being identified with the lesbian community [testing a hypothesis that the client may hold negative beliefs about lesbians].

CLIENT: Well, I don't think that's the case. I do write a monthly article for the gay newspaper. I've also given a good deal of money to the Lesbian Resource Center and have my name identified with that.

THERAPIST: So it's not that you don't like to be around other lesbians [self-correcting through collaboration with the client to better understand the client's perspective].

CLIENT: Well, not in groups, but I wish I had more lesbian friends.

THERAPIST: So do you tend to dislike being around groups of people?

CLIENT: Yes. Well, I can handle a small dinner party, maybe four or five folks. In larger groups, though, I never know what to say. So, I just avoid them.

THERAPIST: So when you tell me you are not into the scene, do you think that you might be afraid of going out to places where there are large groups of people?

CLIENT: Well, yes, that's true. I like the lesbian community. I like gay men. In fact, I like people in general, but I just can't take them all at once. I also haven't ever had an easy time meeting strangers.

THERAPIST: That helps me to understand a little better.

In this exchange, it became clearer to the therapist that the client was not expressing distaste for the gay and lesbian community; rather, she was expressing a fear of groups. The therapist could then begin to assess for social phobia (possibly even panic with agoraphobia) and try to understand the various contexts in which the client felt fear (the situation variables). The client had already indicated her response to such situations, when she stated that she avoided large groups of people. From this brief exchange, the particular consequences of her behavior are not clear, although we can guess that she is having difficulty dating. The therapist would first need to understand more about her particular learning history.

OBJECTIVE MEASURES

Structured interviews and objective measures can be helpful in a behavioral assessment. Some structured interviews are cumbersome for the clinician who often has limited time to make a diagnosis. Researchers use instruments such as the Structured Clinical Interview for DSM-IV Axis I Disorders (First, Spitzer, Gibbon, & Williams, 1996), or the Anxiety Disorders Interview Schedule for DSM-IV (ADIS-IV; DiNardo, Brown, & Barlow, 1994) for ensuring accurate diagnoses in psychotherapy field trials. Clinicians who have not been trained in the use of these measures can review them to make a diagnostic interview comprehensive, if abbreviated. Making an accurate clinical diagnosis can be improved upon over time, and these structured interviews are useful formats for both beginners and experienced clinicians who wish to improve diagnostic skills. For most DSM-IV diagnoses, an empirically supported treatment protocol exists (see Barlow, 2001b). However, in the ongoing process of therapy, as the clinician learns more about the client, changes in diagnosis are appropriate and also help to modify the case conceptualization as needed.

In most clinical settings, briefer measures can be useful in monitoring outcome and refining one's understanding of the patient's problems. After the therapist has conducted an interview and has a general understanding of the client's complaint, he or she can conduct a more fine-grained interview using the behavioral assessment techniques discussed earlier, as well as incorporating questions from the structured interviews to rule out competing diagnoses or comorbid problems. At this point in the assessment, the use of self-report measures can guide both diagnosis and treatment. The Association for Advancement of Behavior Therapy has recently published two volumes that provide superb information about evaluating clients for anxiety disorders (Antony, Orsillo & Roemer, 2001) and depression (Nezu, Ronan, Meadows, & McClure, 2000). These volumes include not only psychometric data on most of the available measures for these disorders but also reprints of several of the inventories clinicians can use with their clients.

Many cognitive-behavioral therapists also rely on scales that can be repeated over time to determine therapeutic effectiveness. The Beck Depression Inventory (BDI; Beck, Ward, Mendelson, Mock, & Erbaugh, 1961) and the BDI—Second Edition (BDI-II; Beck, Steer, & Brown, 1996) are widely used measures and can be administered to a client every session or periodically in the therapy process to assess level of depression. Although the BDI is not used alone as a diagnostic measure, it is helpful once a diagnosis of depression has been determined, because there are cutoffs to indicate whether the client's depression is in the mild, moderate, or severe range. Therefore, over the course of therapy, the BDI can provide an objective measure of client improvement.

A related measure, the Beck Hopelessness Scale (BHS; Beck, & Steer, 1988) is a quick, self-administered scale that measures hopelessness about the future and can be useful in assisting the therapist to manage a suicidal client. If the client is expressing a high degree of hopelessness about the future, he or she may be at greater risk for suicide, or at least prone to suicidal ideation. Low scores on this inventory do not rule out suicidal behavior, however, so therapists must use this and all self-report measures in the context of ongoing assessment and sound clinical management.

There are also useful measures of anxiety. The volume by Antony et al. (2001) includes measures for generalized anxiety, panic and agorophobia, specific phobia, social phobia, acute stress, posttraumatic stress disorder, and obsessive–compulsive disorder. Despite their psychometric validation, therapists should carefully review inventories prior to presentation to any client, so that they may be aware of questions that could be misunderstood by a client as homophobic or heterosexist. It is, in fact, good practice to review all assessment measures used for possible offensive or biased content, because clinicians are not likely to know the sexual orientation of clients prior to the initial interview. The clinician need not utterly rule out the use of a measure because of one or two items, however, especially when an item may suggest an important aspect of the disorder. The Yale–Brown Obsessive–Compulsive Scale (Y-BOCS; Goodman et al., 1989), for example, has three items that could be interpreted as judgmental by a LGB client but are intended to assess obsessions about sexual practices. Many clients with obsessive–compulsive disorder have worries about their sexual behaviors or about sexual identity. These questions are essential in the evaluation of a client presenting with obsessive–compulsive disorder, and it would be foolish for the clinician to fear including them with a LGB client. The questions are also asked by the clinician and can be phrased in a manner that is not offensive or judgmental.

Questionnaires that can easily be used with same-sex couples are more difficult to find than structured interviews. Many measures are clearly written for married couples, and the inclusion of the word "marriage" is offensive to many same-sex couples who are legally barred from marriage in most states. To practice in a culturally sensitive manner with same-sex couples, the therapist must use measures that are not concerned with marriage, and that are gender-neutral (Martell & Land, 2002). One such scale, the Dyadic Adjustment Scale (DAS; Spanier, 1976), is a measure of distress in couple relationships. The scale uses gender-neutral language and assesses areas of conflict for couples, as well as level of commitment and each partner's perception of intimate behaviors. The Conflict Tactics Scale (CTS; Straus, 1979) is an important measure for couples, because it provides screening for domestic violence. This measure is also gender-neutral and can easily be used with same-sex couples.

Throughout the course of therapy, the therapist may make use of clinical manuals or published self-help materials for clients. Therapists should, of course, read any material to review for offensive or invalidating content prior to presenting it to a LGB client. Charts and self-monitoring materials are presented in later chapters that focus on particular disorders. Clinical manuals that include homework materials and self-monitoring tools for clients that contain language suitable for use with sexual-minority clients are also presented in later chapters.

Cognitive-behavioral therapists working with LGB clients have a rich literature of careful assessment on which they can draw to develop meaningful treatment plans with their clients. Behavioral assessment is fundamentally nonjudgmental. The behaviors of interest are those that are problematic for the clients or for significant others in their lives. The therapist works collaboratively with the client to formulate a case conceptualization and to develop treatment goals. Once the therapist has a solid understanding of the behavioral, cognitive, environmental, and affective components of the client's life, he or she can begin to plan interventions that can be tested for effectiveness with the client. We now turn to the basics of treatment that should be included in competent CBT.

Chapter 3

The Basics of Cognitive-Behavioral Therapies

Once a therapist has conducted a behavioral assessment and defined treatment goals, he or she can proceed with treatment, with ongoing assessment of client progress. In this chapter, we present the basics of CBT. The movement in psychology to demonstrate empirically validated treatments has motivated more practitioners to learn about CBT, because many of the treatments that meet criteria for empirical support (Chambless et al., 1998) are cognitive-behavioral methods. Additionally, there has been pressure from the insurance industry for psychotherapists to demonstrate accountability: that treatment is goal focused, and that positive outcomes are being achieved. This chapter primarily serves those readers who do not have a strong background in CBT. However, because our focus is the application to a particular population of people, it may also be helpful to readers who have CBT experience but lack training or experience working with LGB clients. Despite the tendency to speak of CBT as if it were a singular form of therapy, there are actually several theoretical subtypes that fall under the rubric of CBT. Additionally, specific disorders may have specific cognitive-behavioral treatment protocols that can be applied to them. In this chapter, we present some basics of CBT that constitute generally good practice with LGB clients regardless of the specific protocol used for a particular disorder.

COGNITIVE-BEHAVIORAL THERAPY IS A STRUCTURED THERAPY

Behavior therapies have been developed around formulating therapeutic goals for treatment and developing steps to reach these goals. They thus establish clear, long-range therapeutic objectives, as well as a structure within each session. Cognitive therapists are considered competent only when they adhere to this structure (J. S. Beck, 1995).

Accountability for treatment outcomes lies at the heart of CBT and therapists keep track of therapy success by setting goals with clients early on in therapy. CBT is usually a short-term treatment, so treatment goals should be specific and attainable. Treatment usually focuses on the "here and now" rather than on understanding childhood experiences or finding putative reasons in the past for current behavior (Beck, 1976). Goals such as learning assertiveness skills or understanding how to respond to automatic thoughts to stabilize emotions can be achieved relatively quickly. Typically, treatment protocols assume that therapy will last from 12 to 24 weeks. Within this period, therapists must set specific, smaller goals that follow a stepwise process in attaining overall treatment goals. Some presenting problems may call for more than a brief intervention. In such cases, therapists can define long-term goals with clients—such as changing core beliefs or managing personality disorders.

Changing a specific belief or idea can be a short-term, stepwise goal, for example, in treating depression. The therapist helps the client to change stereotyped distorted beliefs to be more balanced or rational (Beck, Rush, Shaw, & Emery, 1979). On the other hand, learning a new skill can be a general treatment goal. In assertiveness training, for example, clients learn to state their needs and desires in an assertive rather than aggressive or passive manner (Alberti & Emmons, 2001).[1]

COGNITIVE-BEHAVIORAL THERAPY IS EMPIRICALLY DERIVED

The treatments available to CBT therapists derive more from empirical observations than from theoretical ideas. Once a treatment has been developed, it is tested in randomized clinical trials (RCTs). Most CBT therapies have specific manuals or protocols that are followed in RCTs. Therapists who work in these trials must demonstrate both competence in and adherence to the protocols to deliver treatment in a uniform way, so that the treatment can be compared to alternative interventions or controls.

COGNITIVE-BEHAVIORAL THERAPY
RELIES ON FUNCTIONAL ANALYSIS

CBT has provided therapists with the understanding that the function of a client's behavior is important in modifying such behavior. In Chapter 2, we described cognitive-behavioral assessment, emphasizing the importance of understanding the antecedents, behaviors, and consequences of behavior in CBT. The functional analysis is essential in fully understanding a client's behavior and in planning interventions.

In CBT, both the designated treatment for a specific disorder and the within-session techniques for evaluating client progress are based on empirical evidence. CBT's emphasis on behavioral analysis and case conceptualization allows the therapist flexibility in using protocols with specific clients. These three principles—that CBT is structured, empirically derived, and relies on a functional analysis—make it a unique form of psychotherapy.

FROM ASSESSMENT TO TREATMENT

Once the therapist has conducted a thorough behavioral assessment and has made a diagnosis, he or she can begin to set treatment goals with the client. As mentioned earlier, there is an emphasis on overall treatment goals, as well as on goals for each session. Diagnostic categories may suggest certain treatment targets—for example, a client with a specific phobia may seek to face a fear; a client suffering from depression may have the goal of becoming more active. The clinician also needs to use the problem list (see Chapter 2) to identify targets for each client. When a client's symptoms meet criteria for a specific DSM-IV disorder, the clinician can use empirically derived protocols for certain disorders. A selection of these protocols is presented later, when we address several specific disorders.

Often, clients come to therapy with vague complaints. They may say they are depressed or anxious all the time. Clients also may believe their problems consist of those that are presented in the popular press. Thus, a client who has recently broken up with a partner may seek therapy because she wishes to be less "codependent." A client who has difficulty meeting people may say that he suffers from "low self-esteem." The therapist needs to determine whether the client meets criteria for a formal diagnosis. The challenge for the CBT therapist is to operationalize the client's ideas about his or her presenting problems, so that treatment targets can be formulated. Furthermore, assessment is not a one-time event in CBT, and the clinician will continually conduct functional analyses to understand better the source and consequence of a client's problem.

Let's take the case of the often seen but frustratingly vague problem of "codependence." Rita came to therapy following a breakup with a partner of 6 years. The two women had lived together for 5 of the 6 years, but during the first year of their relationship, they had dated long-distance, because Rita's partner was in school in another city. Rita suggested that she move to the town in which her girlfriend lived after the first 2 weeks they were together, but her girlfriend told her to keep her good job, and they could see each other on weekends. They saw each other every weekend the first year, with Rita traveling 3 hours each way by car. Rita was 28 when she came to therapy. She had met her girlfriend, Dana, when she was 22 and had just finished college. At that time, she had a very good job but was feeling uncertain about her ability to succeed in a field in which she was a novice just out of college. The therapist asked Rita if Dana had required her to drive down to see her each weekend back then. She replied, "Oh, no. We never talked about it. She was in school, and I had more money for gas. So, I just did it. I wanted to see her so badly."

After Dana graduated from nursing school, she found a job in the city where Rita lived, and the two of them rented a house together. Rita said that their relationship was "blissfully happy" for the first 2 years, but in the third year, they began to have problems. Their sexual life was diminishing, and Dana complained of being bored. Rita said she was perfectly content and could not understand why Dana was unhappy. For the third and fourth year of their relationship, they continued to live together but became increasingly isolated from one another. They purchased an old house together during this time, and Rita began a project of remodeling the home. She and Dana worked together on many of the projects, but they also needed to hire contractors to do plumbing and electrical work. This required that they both take overtime work in their jobs whenever it was available, because they needed to pay for the work to be done. Rita said Dana began to stay out late with friends after work and to spend a great deal of time with one friend in particular. Rita became suspicious of the relationship but didn't say anything for fear of losing Dana. Also, she felt overwhelmed with the responsibility for the remodeling and did not think it was the right time to have any conflict with Dana.

Rita's suspicions were well founded. Dana told her that she had become involved in a relationship with the other woman. Rita said that she was "devastated" by the news and that she had a "breakdown" and didn't eat or sleep for a week. She and Dana continued to live together for the next year, while they finished the remodeling projects that were well under way. Once they completed these projects, they put their house on the market and split the profit. Rita thought that she should have gotten more than Dana, because she had originally put a larger amount of money into the down payment, and she had done all of the wall papering, painting, and even some of the woodwork refinishing, with very little help from Dana.

Hearing the story, the therapist began to hypothesize some of the problems that could become targets for treatment and that needed follow-up. First, several of the situations Rita described suggested that she did not assert herself with Dana, and the therapist wanted to know if this behavior was consistent in other situations, and with other people. Second, Rita apparently made assumptions about Dana that may or may not have been true—for instance, that Dana wanted her to do all of the driving for visits during the first year of their relationship. Third, Rita talked about being uncertain on her job, and the therapist wanted to know if this had improved as she had gained experience, or if it was still a problem for her.

Rita had described herself as "codependent," but the therapist was beginning to think Rita may have lacked assertiveness skills, held faulty beliefs about how much a person needed to give of herself in a relationship, made inaccurate assumptions, or feared conflict. Lumping all of these together under the rubric of "codependence" did nothing to help with the treatment, and it pathologized Rita completely, without suggesting suitable targets for treatment. So the therapist went to work to complete a behavioral analysis of what Rita described, and to develop treatment goals with her.

THERAPIST: Rita, I can tell that you are very upset about this relationship ending. I would like to understand you a little better in terms of how your life is apart from this relationship.

RITA: Is there life apart from this relationship? That's my problem, I'm just so damn dependent on her that I feel like I can't live without her.

THERAPIST: I understand that you believe life isn't worth living without Dana. Have you actually thought of ending your life since the breakup?

RITA: God no. I'm too cowardly.

THERAPIST: I actually think it takes courage to keep going after a loss. Can you tell me what has kept you going?

RITA: Well, I have my job. I actually really like the job and have been given a lot of responsibility. Last month, my boss asked me if I was ready to move into upper management and be in charge of three workgroups instead of just the one I currently supervise.

THERAPIST: You supervise your workgroup?

RITA: Yes, I've been a supervisor for 3½ years. The position of taking over the other teams just opened, because the guy that was doing it before wanted to transfer out of state to be closer to his father, who is ill.

THERAPIST: Can you tell me what it is like to supervise the workgroup?

RITA: Well, most of the people in my group are great. There are five of us in all. Three of the guys are terrific and really do their work. I am one of two women, and I must say it is tough working with the other woman in my group. She's very vindictive and has tried to do a few things behind my back with my boss.

THERAPIST: What did you do in those circumstances?

RITA: Well, it has happened twice. The first time, I was very nice and told her that I was disappointed that she had talked to Hal rather than coming to me. I also told her that, in the future, I wanted her to feel free to talk through any complaints or difficulties she was having. The second time, though, when I found out she had gone over my head because she didn't agree on a decision I had made about one of our vendors, I got really mad. I kept my cool but told her that I was giving her a verbal warning that her behavior was unacceptable as part of a team. I also told her I was willing to entertain her disagreement, but that my decisions were, in some cases, final, and she would need to live with them, because I was the one ultimately responsible for them.

THERAPIST: That is very interesting to me that you handled that situation so directly. When you were telling me about Dana, it sounded like you didn't handle conflict with her in the same way.

RITA: Of course not. I hated conflict with her. I was afraid she'd leave me if we had a fight.

THERAPIST: [using this example to begin to define thoughts and behaviors that might be a focus of treatment] So, you believed that if you fought with her, she would leave you.

RITA: Yes.

THERAPIST: And you just did everything that she wanted.

RITA: Well, mostly, yes.

THERAPIST: Did you do things, even if she hadn't directly asked you to?

RITA: Yes, I·tried to anticipate her needs.

THERAPIST: How did she respond to that?

RITA: Well, she left me for someone else, didn't she?

THERAPIST: Yes, ultimately. But I'm wondering how she responded in specific situations when you would anticipate her needs.

RITA: Well, let me think. I remember one time when we were working on the kitchen. The new appliances were going to be installed, and the cupboards needed to be varnished. We were going to do that ourselves. She had to spend the day at a continuing education conference for her nursing certificate. I thought I'd surprise her. I took a personal day and did the varnishing, so that it would be done by the time she got home.

THERAPIST: And how did she react?

RITA: She was actually a little disappointed. She said that she thought we were going to do it together over the weekend. She also was a little miffed at me for taking the personal day. I thought that was pretty ungrateful.

THERAPIST: So do you think there were times when you assumed that she wanted you to do certain things, and when you did them, she actually was upset with you because that hadn't been what she wanted?

RITA: I suppose so. I guess I really blew it.

THERAPIST: Well, it was a kind gesture you were making. But I wonder if you were doing some of those things to compensate because of your idea that she would leave you, and not because she really wanted you to do them.

RITA: Yeah, that's a good point, because when she told me that she was unhappy and had started dating someone else, she said she "needed someone who could live her own life as well as participate with hers." She basically said I was too clinging.

THERAPIST: It sounds like you did things in the relationship that could feel like clinging to your partner. However, you don't seem very clinging at work. In fact, you sound to me like you are a take-charge kind of person.

RITA: I am, at work. I don't really care about those people. We are all there to do a job.

THERAPIST: Well, if you were 100% "codependent," you would be so at home and at work. So do you think it would be good for us to look at situations like your relationship with Dana, where you think and act in ways that ultimately make life harder for you?

RITA: Sure. I think there are other situations, too. Like with my mother. I kind of act the same way around her, but she doesn't seem to mind. In fact, she expects it.

THERAPIST: That may be one of the places you learned to act this way.

RITA: My dad, who died 9 years ago, was a tyrant. He was the "Shut up and get me a beer" kind of guy. He was great with me but tough on my older brother and my mom. She would always get him the beer.

THERAPIST: So she anticipated his needs. Sort of like you do in your relationships. [Makes a connection for Rita that behaviors learned in the past through observation may now be present in current situations. Learned behaviors can be unlearned.]

RITA: Yes, I think I do that a little.

THERAPIST: It sounds to me like there are three main areas we need to work on. One is to help you recognize and evaluate how useful some of your ideas about relationships are. A second, related area is to look at ideas and beliefs that you have about yourself, and the different ways you act in different situations. We'll try to plan better strategies in those situations where your behavior is getting in the way. Third, I think it would be a good idea to talk about how to deal with the difficult emotions that are present when you need to confront someone that you are very close to. How do those goals sound to you? [In summarizing goals, the therapist works to gain the client's collaboration.]

RITA: They sound like what I need, but I don't even know where to begin.

THERAPIST: Well, we can only work on one at a time, so the first step is to set some priorities for how to go about this.

Note that several things were happening in this interchange. The therapist initially accepted the client's interpretation of her problem as "codependence." There is never a need to argue with a client over terms. In fact, the therapist eventually stated that it seemed that the client was not "100% codependent." The therapist also listened carefully to the client's story and then suggested the idea of three broad categories of behavior to change. Note that the therapist also asked the client for input about these goals and enlisted her agreement with them. The therapist looked at this case from a classic CBT perspective. She began a

functional analysis by assessing the context or situations in which problem behaviors occurred, following the principle that behavior is situation-specific and cannot be assumed to be ubiquitous. The therapist
also questioned the "organismic" variables by asking Rita if she thought
she was trying to compensate for a rule she followed: "If I confront
someone I love, he or she will leave me." Also, the therapist briefly
asked about Rita's family but did not get bogged down in too much hy-
pothesizing, other than to state that she may have developed some of
her problematic behavior in relationships by watching and participating
in her family. The therapist also asked about the consequences of Rita's
behavior in several circumstances. As the sessions continue, the therapist will want to have much more specific descriptions of situations,
thoughts, behaviors, and outcomes. First, however, the therapist needs
to help Rita prioritize her goals.

PRIORITIZING GOALS

Few protocols suggest which therapy goals should take priority. Usually,
the therapist and client collaborate on the matter and come to an agreement on which broad goals to tackle first. In dialectical behavior
therapy (Linehan, 1993a), which is discussed later in the book, certain
behaviors take precedence over others as part of the therapy protocol.
This therapy was developed with suicidal, self-harming women with
borderline personality disorder, and understandably targets self-harm
behaviors before all others. This should be the case with any dangerous
behaviors in which a client may engage. Suicidal behaviors, self-
mutilation, excessive drug or alcohol use, involvement in a physically
abusive relationship, or engagement in illegal activities that could result
in the client having serious trouble with the law should always be prior-
itized as more important. Even perfect CBT therapists can't help a client
if he or she is dead, in a coma, or in prison. So when the therapist
knows of such behaviors or intentions, these should be the first targets
of intervention. Therapists must be aware of their own values in this
process, however, and take care not to impose them on the client. For
example, a client may smoke cigarettes or even marijuana regularly.
Some therapists may disapprove of this behavior or hold strong values
opposing use of unhealthy or illegal substances. However, if an assessment does not demonstrate substance dependence, the client is comfortable with the risk he or she is taking, and there are no other adverse
effects that can clearly be defined, the therapist should allow the client
autonomy in making personal decisions about the issue.[2]

In most cases, the therapist will set priorities in collaboration with the client. He or she should give thought to the types of targets that will make the most impact overall, and suggest that therapy begin with these. A middle-age man sought therapy because he was fearful of driving after having been involved in a serious automobile accident. He also believed that his social life was sorely lacking and that his overwhelming sense of loneliness and isolation were making him depressed. He was best served by increasing his mobility and becoming comfortable driving again, prior to tackling the problems with his social life. In situations in which there is no obvious priority, collaboration between therapist and client is the best road to setting the order of problems to target. In some cases, several target behaviors may be worked on simultaneously.

SESSION STRUCTURE

To varying degrees, CBT therapies have a standard session structure. When a therapist follows a particular treatment protocol, the structure of the session is an important ingredient. Therapists must both stay within a protocol and allow enough flexibility to maintain a good relationship with the client and address client needs that do not fit a protocol exactly (Addis, Hatgis, Soysa, Zaslavsky, & Bourne, 1999). However, therapists who are new to following treatment protocols and adhering to the session-by-session structure are often surprised by the robust nature of such empirically derived protocols. There is a myth that such treatments do not allow adequate creativity or focus on the client to make lasting change. The therapist can indeed be flexible with certain aspects of the structure. For example, therapists may routinely administer questionnaires prior to each therapy session, or periodically, during the course of therapy. It is recommended that therapists monitor client progress throughout, and objective measures are the best way of doing this. However, in some cases, the therapist may choose to use behavioral markers instead, such as the amount of time involved in a repetitive, compulsive activity (with the goal being to see a decrease in times of involvement). If the therapist is using objective measures, it is preferable to leave them for the client to complete prior to the therapy session, so that any notable changes can be discussed as part of the agenda. CBT therapists are expected to set an agenda for each session. Although clients often set agendas simply to discuss certain situations or feelings they've had, it is more productive if the therapist can guide the agenda somewhat, so there is a clear goal that both client and therapist can evaluate. Session agendas are decided with input from the client.

Self-Report Measures

Clients can easily be socialized to complete forms and questionnaires prior to a therapy session. Scales such as the BDI (Beck et al., 1961, 1996) or the Beck Anxiety Inventory (BAI; Beck, Epstein, Brown, & Steer, 1988) can be used as measures of client improvement. Typically, because assessment is a part of treatment, if the person's goals for therapy involve something that can be quantified in the form of a self-report measure, these measures can provide insight into a client's progress and/or his or her impediments to progress. A simple rationale to present to clients is that problems in life often feel unrelenting. When one is depressed or anxious, it may seem that there is no change in the intensity. Completing a self-report questionnaire that asks the client to rate how he or she felt over the previous week can provide a picture of mood fluctuations.[3]

The Agenda

Setting a session agenda is the only way to focus on one or two problems with the client. Because many clients present with multiple issues and very little will be resolved unless problems are addressed systematically, the therapist has to take primary responsibility for setting the agenda for each session. Setting agendas promotes change and enhances treatment outcome, and provides permission for the therapist to gently bring the client back to topic if he or she strays. Likewise, setting an agenda in every session keeps the therapist on track. Deviating from an agenda is not always countertherapeutic, but any change from an agreed-upon agenda should be discussed briefly with the client first.

Recall that there were three broad goals discussed in the case of Rita. She and her therapist had agreed that the first priority was her discomfort in highly charged emotional encounters with individuals with whom she was very close. They made this a priority, because Rita said that she had great difficulty engaging in negative encounters with lovers, friends, and family. The therapist also believed that some of the beliefs and ideas that were dysfunctional for Rita would be encountered in this process and could be addressed simultaneously. With the overall goal in place, the therapist needed to get specific details from Rita. They had planned to talk about any difficulty Rita might have had in the week between therapy sessions. Still, the therapist collaborated with Rita to set a session agenda. Keep in mind that setting the agenda early in the session also reduces the likelihood that the client will bring up

important topics at the very end of the session, when there is not time
to address them.

THERAPIST: I can see from your depression inventory that you are feeling a little better this week than when you first came in. Would you
say that is accurate with your experience?

RITA: Yes, I think that talking to you last week helped a little.

THERAPIST: Good. Last week, we decided to begin working on your discomfort with negative interactions with people you care about
deeply. That is a fairly large goal. So you were going to try to be
aware of any examples of the problem that occurred during the
week for us to talk about. Did anything come up that we should put
on our agenda to discuss today?

RITA: Well, it wasn't very intense, but I did have a situation with my
friend Ken that I think might be an example.

THERAPIST: So we should talk about the situation with Ken. Was there
anything specific about that situation?

RITA: Do you want me to tell you what happened?

THERAPIST: I do, but before you do that, I just want to know if we
should be focusing on anything in particular in the interaction.

RITA: No, I think the whole situation is illustrative of what I typically
do.

THERAPIST: Would you like to talk about anything else today, or do you
think that this item will require our whole session?

RITA: I'd like to talk a little more about Dana.

THERAPIST: Is there something specific about Dana that you'd like to
discuss?

RITA: I've just been thinking about her a lot, and about how I really
screwed up that relationship. I've been thinking about her happily
involved in a new relationship, while I feel lousy and have had to
start therapy because of this.

THERAPIST: Then, we should talk about how you feel when you think
about Dana's circumstances compared to your own?

RITA: Yes, I think that would be good.

THERAPIST: Do you think that you will feel like you got what you
wanted from this session, if we cover these two items?

RITA: I think so, yes.

THERAPIST: Shall we begin with the situation with Ken or with Dana?

RITA: Since it's on my mind, let's talk about Dana. That is really what is bothering me.

THERAPIST: Fine. We'll just make sure we leave time to talk about what happened with Ken.

Some therapists (e.g., J. S. Beck, 1995) recommend that specific times be assigned to each item on the agenda. Therapists may choose to do this, but it is a matter of style. Setting the agenda should take place within the first 5–10 minutes of the session. Within this time, the therapist can prioritize items with the client and set times, if desired. The important idea is always to agree on the topic for discussion with the client at the beginning of each therapy session. If the client has had an assignment between sessions (see below), it needs to be placed on the agenda. Likewise, if there have been incidences of dangerous or harmful behaviors on the part of the client, these need to take precedence over other agenda items.

The Body of the Session

There are many CBT techniques from which a therapist can choose to address specific client problems. Table 3.1 provides a list of selected techniques, with references for further reading. We discuss several treatments in detail in later chapters of the book. Generally, CBT can be viewed as a therapy with several branches. Some practitioners emphasize the behavioral aspects of treatment and may use cognitive components as part of therapy but view cognition as behavior, and do not necessarily subscribe to the cognitive theory of emotional disorders. This branch of CBT includes the radical behaviorists (those who are heavily influenced by the work of B. F. Skinner), whose work is typically referred to as behavior modification or applied behavior analysis. Related, but with a slightly different emphasis, are the behavior therapists [those who predominantly use techniques such as Wolpe's (1982) systematic desensitization], who focus on the treatment of problems seen more often by clinicians in outpatient settings.

Of the cognitive therapists, three major schools of thought predominate within this branch: rational–emotive therapy, cognitive therapy, and cognitive constructivism.[4]

With the exception of the most orthodox researchers and practitioners of these various configurations of CBT, most professionals combine approaches. So the combination of the terms "cognitive" and "behavioral" has been justified. There is certainly collegial sparring over

TABLE 3.1. Cognitive-Behavioral Techniques, with References for Further Study

Technique	Description	Reference(s)
Anxiety management training	Teaches the client regarding specific situations. When anxious imagery causes the client to indicate high anxiety, the client then practices relaxation until anxiety is reduced. The client alternates between anxiety imagery and relaxation.	Suinn (1990)
Assertiveness training	Teaches clients to specify desires and needs using "minimally effective" responses to assert their position. Useful for either unassertive or overly aggressive clients.	Alberti & Emmons (2001)
Behavioral activation	Increases activity for depressed or passive clients by using activity scheduling and other techniques.	Martell, Addis, & Jacobson (2001)
Behavior rehearsal	Simulates real-life situations during the therapeutic hour, allowing client to practice desired behaviors.	Goldfried & Davison (1976/1994, Ch. 7)
Communication skills training	Used in couple therapy to help couples talk about feelings and problems in a manner that resolves rather than exacerbates problems.	Jacobson & Margolin (1979)
Downward arrow	Therapist solicits a thought from client regarding a particular situation and asks client, "If this is true, what does this mean about you, or your life?" Therapist and client move "downard," until they uncover the client's underlying assumptions.	J. S. Beck (1995).
Exposure	Used in many treatments for anxiety. Client faces fear stimuli without resorting to escape or avoidance maneuvers. Exposure can be done in real life (*in vivo*) or using imagery.	Foa & Goldstein (1978)
Flooding	Similar to exposure, but the client is "flooded" with feared stimuli, until anxiety peaks and then subsides.	Goldfried & Davison (1976/1994, Ch. 6)
Finding alternatives	In cognitive therapy, client reviews all possible options and alternatives to see for either interpreting a situation or resolving a problem.	J. S. Beck (1995)
Labeling distortions	A cognitive therapy technique that teaches the client to recognize and label particular distortions in thinking that can lead to problems with interpretation of events.	Burns (1980/1999)

(*continued*)

TABLE 3.1. (*continued*)

Technique	Description	Reference(s)
Mastery/pleasure ratings	Clients use activity chart (see "Behavioral activation") and rates amount of mastery or pleasure that they derive from activity.	J. S. Beck (1995)
Opposite action	Client is encouraged to engage in behavior that would be counterintuitive or opposite to what he or she may feel at the time (e.g., when feeling very angry, say something kind or decent).	Linehan (1993b)
Panic control therapy	Utilizes various cognitive and behavioral techniques to treat panic and agoraphobia, including interoceptive exposure, wherein therapist teaches client to engage in activities in session that create feelings that lead to panic, allowing the client to reinterpret interoceptive cues.	Craske, Barlow, & Meadows (2000)
Problem-solving training	Teaches a step approach of orienting to the problem, problem definition, generation of alternatives, decision making, and solution implementation and verification of results.	D'Zurilla & Nezu (1982)
Relaxation training	Teaches client to relax muscles to condition a relaxation response to counter tension. Uses imagery, music, and other stimuli to assist in acquiring response.	Goldfried & Davison (1976/1994, Ch. 5)
Rational restructuring	Used in Beck's cognitive therapy and rational–emotive behavior therapy of Ellis. Teaches client to identify irrational, distorted, or maladaptive beliefs, question the evidence for the belief, and generate alternative responses.	J. S. Beck (1995) Ellis & Harper (1997)
Successive approximation (also known as guided task assignments)	Client and therapist collaborate in developing a plan for the client to engage in steps that approximate an ultimate goal, to allow the client to have success at each step along the way to the goal.	J. S. Beck (1995)
Three-column technique	Client collects automatic thoughts and lists the situation in which thought occurred, the automatic thought, and the associated feelings.	Schuyler (1991)
Thought Record	Expands on the three-column technique, with columns to record alternative responses to the automatic thought, and behavioral or emotional outcomes of changing the thought.	Beck, Rush, Shaw, & Emery (1979)

whether the cognitive aspects of behavior therapy are necessary, or whether cognition is, in fact, simply behavior that is private (a position proposed earlier in this book). Our example of Rita demonstrates how the therapist draws from both cognitive and behavioral techniques in addressing the problems listed for the session agenda. Rita first wanted to talk about thinking about Dana, her ex-partner, and how such thoughts made her feel depressed. Such a problem can be addressed in several ways. After getting more detail, the therapist decided to approach this by having Rita evaluate the idea that she had "screwed up" and also discuss reducing the amount of time that Rita spent thinking about Dana.

THERAPIST: Do you think that you were responsible for your relationship with Dana ending?

RITA: Ultimately, she was the one who ended the relationship, but I think that I pushed her away.

THERAPIST: How did you do that?

RITA: I was too clinging. I never did what I wanted to do and always acquiesced to her. She ultimately got bored with me.

THERAPIST: So you think that the relationship ended because you were too submissive?

RITA: Not exactly. I really cared about her, but probably too much. In general, I'm pretty good at standing up for myself. At work, for example, I usually take charge of things, but not always, as you'll see when we talk about Ken. Still, with Dana, I didn't really care about my needs. In fact, her needs felt like my needs. I was happy to do what she wanted, because I enjoyed spending time with her.

THERAPIST: Do you have specific interests that you needed to ignore so you could do the things that Dana wanted?

RITA: No. I am pretty flexible. Dana and I really enjoyed the same things. We went to baseball games, liked the same television shows, and occasionally saw plays or the ballet. She took the lead in planning some of the events, but I was always glad to go along. When it came to the· house, we agreed on what we wanted changed. I think I made the mistake of trying to surprise her with getting work done, not realizing that she wanted to do the work as well.

THERAPIST: Are you referring to the time you finished the kitchen cabinets while she was away?

RITA: Yes. That was pretty stupid of me.

THERAPIST: So far, you are saying that it was not important to you what you and Dana did, because you enjoyed the activities. Also, you allowed Dana to make plans, because you did not have strong preferences. Did Dana ever complain to you about this?

RITA: Not that I remember. We just got more distant over time.

THERAPIST: Did the two of you ever talk about the growing distance?

RITA: Not really. We had a few discussions about sex. I would try to initiate, and she would usually push me away. She stopped initiating, and we eventually stopped having sex. I tried to bring it up a few times, but we just got into an argument, so I let it drop.

THERAPIST: Do you see that you actually did try to initiate activity, but your actions weren't reciprocated? This seems to have been the case both with initiating sex and with conversation about the sexual problems. Is it possible that you tried to initiate other activities and that Dana did not follow your lead?

RITA: Perhaps. I can't remember many instances of that. I suppose I did occasionally state my preferences. I wasn't a total doormat.

THERAPIST: So you weren't a total doormat, and Dana never told you that she was unhappy with the way the two of you made decisions.

RITA: Well, I knew she was pissed about the cabinets.

THERAPIST: Yes, so there were a few instances when she expressed her displeasure.

RITA: Sure.

THERAPIST: When you think about the times you tried to initiate, what does that tell you about your behavior in your relationship?

RITA: I suppose that I didn't always just acquiesce. I actually stood up for myself at times. Also, when you point out that she never told me she was unhappy about how I let her make most of the decisions, it makes me think that I am not the only one responsible for our problems.

THERAPIST: The thought that you are not solely responsible for your problems with Dana appears to contradict the idea that you screwed up, doesn't it?

RITA: At least, that I was the only one who screwed up.

THERAPIST: If you were to remind yourself that Dana also had a hand in the problems of your relationship, how do you think that would make you feel?

RITA: I'd still feel sad about it all ending. Perhaps I'd feel a little angry with her. I think that I wouldn't feel so guilty. It also gives me hope that I'm not just a pushover in relationships.

THERAPIST: So although you still feel sad, and even a little angry, you also feel less guilty and a little hopeful. Do you think that trying to evaluate some of these thoughts like "I screwed up" will help you to feel a little better?

RITA: I think it will help a little.

THERAPIST: Good. We'll talk more about how to challenge and evaluate thoughts as we continue our work.

In this exchange, the therapist used Socratic questioning to help Rita evaluate her initial thought and arrive at a different conclusion. The reasoning behind this intervention is that Rita's thought, "I screwed up," places all the responsibility on her and is an overgeneralized idea. Rarely is there only one responsible party in a problematic relationship, so the therapist was confident that there would have been examples of Dana's misbehavior. The therapist also relied on the fact that people do not act in only one way in all situations at all times. Therefore, questioning the idea that Rita's "screw-up" indicated something about her character was justified. The therapist planned to teach Rita to conduct this type of analysis of her thinking and use written thought records (Beck et al., 1979) to do so.

The problem under discussion was not just faulty thinking. Whenever a person engages in one type of behavior, it precludes their engaging in another type. In this case, Rita was spending time ruminating about being to blame for the loss of her past relationship. Although this is typical of one who is grieving, it does not help the person to move forward in life. People often talk about "putting relationships behind them and moving on," but they try to do so by mentally playing out various scenes from the relationship over and over again. Behavior therapists do not simply talk with clients about moving forward or working through problems, they teach them how to do so.

THERAPIST: I'm curious as to how much time you spent thinking about Dana this past week.

RITA: Oh, I was thinking about her just about every night.

THERAPIST: Can you tell me the circumstances? Did you think about her when you were with friends or alone, for example?

RITA: I was alone. I pretty much kept my mind on my work during the day. In fact, I don't think I thought about her at all during the day.

Then, when I was driving home, I would think about her. It was downhill from there.

THERAPIST: Did this happen every evening?

RITA: Just about.

THERAPIST: What about the evenings when this did not happen?

RITA: Well, on Friday, I was invited to go out to a movie with my friends Kim and Nancy. We saw *Shakespeare in Love*, which I was looking forward to, because I have really liked Tom Stoppard's plays.

THERAPIST: Did the movie make you think about Dana?

RITA: No, interestingly. I was amused by the play on actual Shakespearean quotes. It was really engaging.

THERAPIST: Were there other times when you weren't thinking about Dana?

RITA: On Saturday morning, when I was grocery shopping. I love the store I go to and usually find shopping relaxing.

THERAPIST: What were you doing when you were thinking about Dana?

RITA: Either just sitting around the house or staring at the television set. I called a couple of friends but just talked about Dana. In fact, one of my friends had just seen Dana and her new girlfriend, so that made me feel really miserable.

THERAPIST: Do you see a pattern here?

RITA: Well, yes. When I'm doing something other than sitting around or talking to friends about Dana, I actually don't think about her very much.

THERAPIST: Do you remember feeling any differently when you weren't thinking about Dana?

RITA: Oh, yes. I was quite content when I was not thinking about her.

THERAPIST: Do you think it would be helpful to try to develop a plan to spend less time thinking about her?

RITA: I don't really know how to do that.

THERAPIST: Well, if you were engaged in other activities and thought about her less, perhaps you could try to think of some alternatives to sitting around the house or talking to friends about her.

RITA: You mean, like talking to friends about something going on in their lives for a change?

THERAPIST: Exactly.

RITA: Well, it's worth a try.

The two interventions chosen by the therapist show how cognitive and behavioral techniques can be interwoven throughout a therapy session. Much of the therapeutic work in CBT, however, takes place outside of the therapy session. Accordingly, an important aspect of the structure of the CBT session is planning for between-session work.[5]

Homework Assignments

Nearly all CBT therapies rely on between-session homework as an important aspect of the treatment. The only way to transfer skills learned in the therapy session to real life is for the client to practice the skills outside of the therapist's office. Constant practice also increases a client's ability to apply skills in a variety of situations. Assigning between-session homework also allows clients to become aware of situations in which they have difficulty applying the skills. These difficulties are then discussed in future sessions, and solutions developed. Homework assignments should, of course, naturally follow from the therapy session. The therapist should collaborate with the client to ensure that the client understands and is on board with the assignment. If the client does not understand or think an assignment is reasonable, he or she is unlikely to try to complete it. Beck et al. (1979) suggest that the manner in which the therapist assigns and reviews homework determines whether therapeutic collaboration is increased or decreased. Therefore, clients should have input into the assignment. The therapist should ensure that clients understand what is expected of them in the assignment, and anticipate potential problems that clients may have in completing the assignment (see J. S. Beck, 1995).

Rita was given two homework assignments. The first was to record any automatic thoughts related to feeling distressed, and to record her feelings. Therapists can use automatic thought records (Beck et al., 1979) or the triple-column technique (Schuyler, 1991) of having clients write the situation, thought, and feeling. Initially, clients are asked to record automatic thoughts, and the therapist helps them to formulate alternative responses to the thoughts in session. Rita's therapist also had her write a list of activities in which she could engage that would be an alternative to thinking about Dana. Once the list was completed, she was to try to engage in the activity and observe whether she was thinking about Dana less as the week went on. Homework assignments are discussed further in chapters on treatment for specific disorders.

Feedback

Throughout the therapy session, client feedback is elicited. In CBT, clients and therapists both take an active role. The client is asked for input into the agenda for the session and for between-session work. The end of the session is also a good time to ask the client for feedback. He or she can briefly be asked to comment on the pacing of the session, relevance of the material covered, whether the session was helpful, and whether there are things that should be changed in future sessions. By soliciting feedback from the client, the therapist can later make modifications to treatment as appropriate, or explain when a modification would not be appropriate and attempt to help the client understand the importance of particular interventions.

COURSE OF TREATMENT

In CBT, as in any treatment, the course of therapy begins with establishing a good therapeutic relationship. This is done during the initial assessment phase. The collaborative nature of CBT is ideally suited to building a strong relationship. Because the therapist and client work together as a team, the client is also given a share of the responsibility for the outcome of the treatment. There is no set length of treatment in CBT. Outcome studies show CBT interventions lasting for as few as 10 and as many as 24 therapy sessions. In cases in which there are multiple targets, or if there is an Axis II disorder, therapy may take significantly longer. The client's self-report of progress, as well as behavioral markers, or criteria, set for objective measures determine when treatment has been successful and termination is appropriate. It is also useful to discuss treatment progress with the client periodically throughout therapy, so that changes can be made if treatment is not successful. CBT is not a panacea, and in cases in which there is not demonstrable success, the client can be counseled regarding further steps to take, such as referral for medication evaluations.

Chapter 4

Treating Depression

Downward Spiral

Rick lost his partner, Anthony, in December 1993. Anthony had died of complications due to AIDS. His illness was long and difficult, and just prior to his death, he had required hospice care away from their home. Rick felt guilty leaving Anthony alone in hospice, while he attended to his own work and home duties. Rick died at the hospice 2 weeks after his initial admission. At first, Rick tried to keep their house exactly as it had been when Anthony was alive; then, after about 6 months, his friends told him that he needed to get rid of some of Anthony's things. Rick wore most of Anthony's clothing, because they were the same size, but there were old financial records and other things cluttering up the home office that were no longer necessary to keep. Over the months following Anthony's death, Rick became less concerned about maintaining the house. He let the grass in the yard grow and devoted most of his free time away from work to watching videos from a collection of 1940s movies, or watching home movies of trips abroad that he had taken with Anthony. He stopped calling most of his friends and refused 90% of the invitations to join friends for dinners or other recreational activities. Two of his friends helped him to clear his house of Anthony's unnecessary belongings. They had hoped that Rick would begin to reengage with the world. However, this did not happen.

Several years went by, and Rick's emotions and behaviors became increasingly restricted. He could identify feeling bored and sad. Occasionally, he found himself feeling frustrated about this or that. He believed that the best part of his life was over now that Anthony was gone, and he remained at home, with only minimal social interaction. He had not gone out with his friends for over 1½ years; he had stopped exercising at the gym and had lost muscle mass. Rick had no appetite for months at a time and forced himself to eat—mostly cold cereal or eggs. He did have short periods of time, weeks at most, when he felt better. On two occasions, he actually accepted offers for dates with two different men. He went on three dates with one of the men, and they were sexual on their second date. In general, however, Rick was not interested in sex or men.

The only activity that he consistently kept up with was feeding and walking his dog. Sadie was an energetic, 60-pound Labrador retriever, who became very destructive around the house if she was not taken for at least a six-block walk once a day. Making sure that Sadie was well looked after became Rick's primary task. He missed a day of work nearly once a month, because he did not feel like leaving his bed, and he wanted to watch home movies. His boss had been tolerant for the first year after Anthony's death, but because Rick's frequent absenteeism continued well over 2 years, his boss's tolerance was wearing thin. Rick was in danger of losing his job; he had received late fees on his credit card bills and had been threatened with having his electricity turned off, because he was late paying the bill. He had avoided returning so many of his friends' calls that they had ceased calling altogether. Only one of his friends, Terri, continued to make attempts to stay in contact, in spite of month-long periods of not hearing from Rick. Terri convinced Rick that he needed professional help. Two and one-half years after Anthony's death, Rick agreed to seek help from a therapist.

FAULTY BELIEFS

Caroline sought therapy 8 months after leaving a high-paying job and becoming unemployed. She had relocated to a larger city from the small town, where she attended graduate school, to take a job as a systems analyst. Her employer had paid for her to relocate and helped her to find a small house to rent. She had been excited about working for this company, because its equal opportunity policies included sexual orientation, and the company marketed itself as seeking diversity in employees. Caroline thought she would feel comfortable at this company. This proved to be true.

Unfortunately, however, her supervisor, another lesbian woman, was not as welcoming to Caroline. Her supervisor gave her very little help or advice early in her employment, and as projects got behind schedule, she implied that Caroline was not doing an adequate job. Caroline felt betrayed by this woman and complained to the human resources department. This did her little good. Human resources suggested to Caroline that she look for openings elsewhere in the company, but her supervisor needed to release her to take another job. Instead, her supervisor gave her a marginal, 6-month evaluation that nearly guaranteed that Caroline would not find another job within the company. She thought of writing a rebuttal in her employee file, but she began doubting herself.

This had been her first job out of graduate school. Although she had been a good student, the constant criticism over the past 6 months made her wonder whether she was incompetent at her work when faced with real-world problems. It didn't help that her closest friend in this new city was transferred out of state for a job that she could not pass up. Caroline had one male friend from work but was afraid to get him embroiled in her problems. She had also dated a woman, Charlene, briefly, but broke off the relationship when things went badly at work, believing that her pessimistic attitude and constant blue mood would just bring Charlene down.

Caroline started to think that she was incompetent at life in general. She regretted her decision to move and take this job. She looked in the mirror and saw a protruding nose and bad skin, and thought, "How can anyone waste their time on me?" She thought about her desire to someday settle down and have children, then told herself, "Yeah, right, the kid will already have to deal with having me as a mother, let alone dealing with the stigma of having two moms."

When her company announced that layoffs were forthcoming, Caroline knew that this was likely the end for her. So she spoke with the woman in human resources and volunteered to be on the list for people taking voluntary layoffs, which would still allow her to receive unemployment benefits. Her supervisor did not argue and seemed, in Caroline's eyes, pleased to be rid of her.

OVERVIEW OF DEPRESSION

Depression affects nearly 18 million people in the United States alone (Schrof & Shultz, 1999). Depression has been called the "common cold" of behavioral disorders and is seen routinely by clinicians (Burns, 1980/1999). Gay men and lesbian women are more likely to suffer from depression than their heterosexual counterparts (Cochran & Mays, 2000). Although data do not provide reasons for this, researchers have speculated that this is the case because of the impact of discrimination toward and negative societal views about LGB people rather than something inherently "depressing" about being LGB individuals. Treatments for depression have been developed by cognitive-behavioral researchers for over four decades (Beck et al., 1979; Ferster, 1973; Lewinsohn, Youngren, & Grosscup, 1979), and CBT is considered an empirically validated treatment for depression (Chambless et al., 1998).

The cases of Rick and Caroline are typical examples of depression, although they experience depression somewhat differently. This fact emphasizes the need for a good case conceptualization. Although the behavioral activation components of CBT (Lewinsohn et al., 1979) have been shown to be as effective as the full cognitive therapy package (Jacobson et al., 1996), and have been developed into a stand-alone treatment (Martell et al., 2001), in most cases, clinicians utilize both behavioral and cognitive interventions according to the case conceptualization.

In Rick's case, the most outstanding feature of his depression was withdrawal from the world and restriction of activity. Grief is an expected reaction to the death of a loved one. However, when the symptoms of normal grieving, such as intense feelings of sadness, loss of appetite, social isolation, and loss of interest in normal activities, continue as long as they had in Rick's case, a diagnosis of major depressive disorder (MDD) is warranted. Rick's treatment is presented to demonstrate *behavioral* techniques used in treating depression, because the primary treatment for symptoms of lack of interest and inactivity is behavioral activation. In Caroline's case, she had begun seriously to doubt her own abilities and held numerous negative beliefs about herself that were overgeneralized and connected with the onset of her depression. Caroline's case demonstrates *cognitive* interventions. Readers should note that these two cases are not radically distinct from one another, however. Rick often engaged in negative thinking and ruminating about his loss, and believed that his life could not improve, and Caroline's activities were restricted. Hence, therapists need to consider using all interventions available in treating a client. The two cases are presented separately here to demonstrate the robust nature of both behavioral and cognitive techniques.

CASE CONCEPTUALIZATION

Earlier, we presented techniques for cognitive-behavioral case formulation (Persons, 1989; Turkat, 1985). It is important to utilize these techniques to develop a treatment plan with depressed clients. During the initial session following a diagnostic interview, the therapist needs to gather information to generate a problem list (Persons, 1989) and to ascertain the client's beliefs about his or her depression (Addis & Jacobson, 1996). In addition to contributing to case conceptualization, these techniques assist in forming a collaborative relationship.

In Rick's case, he attributed his depressed mood to Anthony's death. He told his therapist, "Life just hasn't seemed worth living. I lost

Anthony, and also several other good friends. My network is gone, so why bother getting up? I'd kill myself except that I feel like I have an obligation to stay alive as long as I can, given that so many guys I loved didn't get that chance." After the initial interview, Rick's therapist had generated the following problem list:

Hopelessness
Markedly decreased activities
Social isolation
Poor performance at work
Truancy from work
Neglect of proper nutrition

Caroline attributed her depression to her own inadequacy. She took responsibility for her misfortunes in life and for feeling badly. Caroline told her therapist, "I want to feel better, but I don't really see why I should or what can help. I'm just not going to get ahead in life. Who would want either to hire me or date me? I feel ashamed of myself for being so weak. I'm just not able to do anything right." The outstanding feature of Caroline's depression was her negative thinking. Her problem list consisted of the following:

Unemployment
Hopelessness
Negative beliefs about self
Negative predictions about the future
Social isolation

TREATMENT

Both these clients felt hopeless. The combination of negative life events, and particularly in Caroline's case, negative ideas about herself, and the negative behavioral reactions that deepened their problems had left them expecting that the future was going to be bleak. The therapist used the Beck Depression Inventory (BDI) and the Beck Hopelessness Scale (BHS; Beck, 1978; Beck & Steer, 1988) to assess change in both depression and hopelessness during therapy. These scales were given to the clients at the beginning of each session. During the initial interview, Rick's BDI score was 36, and his BHS score was 18, meaning that he endorsed nearly all of the items associated with hopeless beliefs. Caroline's BDI score was 40, and her BHS score was 15 during the initial session.

Collaboration between therapist and client is a hallmark of CBT. It is therefore important to bring the client "on board" with the case conceptualization, so that future treatment interventions will make sense. Clients who understand the rationale for doing various homework assignments will be more likely to comply with treatment recommendations. It is helpful to provide reading material to clients in the first session that orients them to the treatment rationale used. A brief treatment rationale for behavioral activation is provided in Martell et al. (2001). Cognitive therapy treatment rationales can be found in J. S. Beck (1995), as well as Greenberger and Padesky (1995). Preprinted pamphlets can be obtained from the Beck Institute for Cognitive Therapy and Research or from the Association for Advancement of Behavior Therapy (see Appendix I).

Once clients have read a brief description of the cognitive-behavioral model, the therapist should make sure that the model is explained in relation to the client's situation. This is how treatments designed with the use of group treatment studies become individualized for particular clients. The basic idea presented to clients from a behavioral perspective is that depression follows a combination of life events or environmental factors and individual vulnerabilities. Characteristic symptoms of depression, such as lethargy and fatigue, decreased interest in activities, and changes in appetite, result in the client decreasing his or her activity level, and, in a sense, retreating from the world. Such retreat or avoidance behaviors bring temporary relief for the client's distress but become secondary problems themselves, because they keep the client in a cycle of inertia, negative rumination, and avoidance that brings him or her out of contact with possible positive reinforcers. For example, in Rick's case, the environmental precursors to his depression were obvious to him. He experienced his life as completely different following Anthony's death and the subsequent deaths of other friends. His subsequent withdrawal and avoidance led to further reduction in reinforcement and exacerbated his depression.

During the discussion of the case conceptualization with Rick, the therapist listed the life events on a white board (see Martell et al., 2001, for detailed descriptions of presenting case conceptualizations to clients).

THERAPIST: Rick, what do you see when you look at these life events that I've listed here?

RICK: I see a crappy life with a lot of losses.

THERAPIST: I, too, see a lot of loss. Do you think there are other life events we should list that may have contributed to your depression?

RICK: How about being gay in the 1970s and 1980s!

THERAPIST: I don't follow you.

RICK: Well, what a hell of a time to come out, fall in love, and all that crap. I came out and AIDS came in.

THERAPIST: So perhaps we should write "AIDS epidemic" as one of the life events, would you agree? [Notice how the therapist does not argue about Rick's overgeneralized negativity regarding being gay during this particular historical period, but takes as truth what Rick is saying and collaborates by adding the significant event to the list of life events.]

RICK: Yeah, that certainly has been significant. I bet that if there hadn't been AIDS, and if so many guys that I loved hadn't gotten sick and died, I wouldn't be depressed. I certainly wasn't before Anthony died.

THERAPIST: So these life events have led to life being less rewarding . . .

RICK: To put it mildly.

THERAPIST: Yes, I suppose I am putting it mildly. How might you put it?

RICK: It led to life sucking.

THERAPIST: Well, I know it feels like life sucks, and there hasn't been much positive in your life for the past few years, but I wonder whether it is just the life events or the fact that you are depressed as a result that makes life feel like it sucks.

RICK: Could be either, I guess.

THERAPIST: So when life is less rewarding, or even when life "sucks," people usually try to do something to cope with that. You have become less involved in the world. I think that probably felt normal for you.

RICK: I just haven't really cared about anything anymore.

THERAPIST: That is what you are coming here for. I'd like to help change that. Let me write down some of the ways I think you've been trying to cope with feeling so depressed. (*Returns to writing on the white board, making a list to the right of the word "depression" including the problems from the problem list.*) It is understandable that you would isolate yourself, stay home from work, and so on, when you feel as depressed as you do. However, the problem is that these behaviors don't ultimately make you feel any better, do they?

RICK: No, I guess they keep me stuck.

THERAPIST: Yes, it is as if doing this comes back around on you and may even make your depression worse. It is a cycle that you are in fact stuck in. Our job here is to try to break the cycle. In order to do that, we need to work with these secondary problem behaviors. That means that our initial task is to help you to engage in your life again.

RICK: I understand that. I can't imagine how.

THERAPIST: If you could have done this on your own, you would have. So we need to work together to help you to do the things that you currently cannot imagine.

In this dialogue, the therapist presents a behavioral model to the client and suggests that treatment will consist of the client changing behaviors that exacerbate depression. However, the therapist includes Rick in the discussion, so that Rick is a part of the formulation. This increases the likelihood that Rick will comply with homework and other therapist recommendations. The therapist does not in any way imply that there is nothing to be depressed about but simply describes the negative cycle that intensifies the effects of the life events. Behavior change cannot be forced on a client, especially one who is depressed and passive. Rick has begun to accept the need to change and is now ready to work with his therapist to learn the steps to do so.

BEHAVIORAL TECHNIQUES

Both behavioral and cognitive techniques are incorporated in CBT for depression. As we have discussed, some cases may warrant use of behavioral rather than cognitive techniques. Indeed, the behavioral components of CBT have been used exclusively in some treatments (Martell et al., 2001). Several techniques that fall in the behavioral category were useful in Rick's treatment.

Behavioral Activation

From the earliest behavioral conception, depression was seen as resulting from low rates of reinforcement or high rates of punishment. Ferster (1973) suggested that individuals respond to contingencies of reinforcement in such a way that their behavior demonstrates what would be diagnosed as depression. In this model, individuals have low rates of positive reinforcement that lead to the development of depression. Lewinsohn et al. (1979) took Ferster's theoretical model and developed a treatment of behavioral activation that was the first behavioral treatment for depression. Using an assessment tool called the Pleasant Events Schedule (MacPillamy & Lewinsohn, 1982), they assessed low levels of self-reported pleasant activities in individuals who subsequently were diagnosed as having a major depressive episode. Their treatment consisted of activity scheduling to increase the number of pleasant events engaged in over a discrete period of time to help mitigate the negative effects of depression.

Although life events have been implicated as precursors to depressive episodes in a number of cases, logic would suggest that there could not possibly be a one-to-one correlation between negative life events and depression. If depression were a direct result of an individual experiencing negative life events, nearly everybody would be depressed. But a majority of individuals experience life problems without developing significant psychopathology. Ferster's behavioral description of reinforcement patterns may provide a key to some of the behavioral history that renders certain individuals vulnerable to depression, while others are not. Furthermore, in later depressed clients, family coping patterns during childhood may be modeled that serve to develop styles of coping that are passive and less functional (Hammen, 1999). Biological factors may also come into play, although there is little evidence that depression per se is directly inherited (Valenstein, 1998).

From a purely behavioral perspective, depressive symptoms, in much the same manner as anxiety symptoms, are maintained by avoidance behaviors (Jacobson, Martell, & Dimidjian, 2001; Martell et al., 2001). The secondary problem behaviors that Rick's therapist recognized are considered avoidance behaviors, because Rick was trying to escape or temporarily alleviate distress by staying away from people, work, and so forth. Ferster (1973) described behaviors such as complaining as avoidance behavior. In other words, because complaining about problems brings temporary relief, or may reduce distress by getting attention from significant others or professional helpers, the behavior basically serves the function of allowing the individual to avoid the negative feelings or life events he or she is experiencing. Avoidance is perpetuated because of the negative reinforcement of temporary reduction of emotional distress (e.g., relief from anxiety, escape from feelings of despair).

Rick's treatment began with behavioral activation (BA) to break the pattern of inertia that had developed after Anthony's death. The first, necessary intervention in BA is to have a good understanding of the client's life during the week. This is the process called behavioral analysis. Clients are asked to record their activities and moods during the week. Figure 4.1 is an example of an activity chart that can be used for several purposes (Martell et al., 2001). Activity charts can be used to assess

Please record the following information in the boxes below: What were you doing? If you were with other people, please note. How were you feeling? Please rate the intensity of the feeling on a 0 (*not at all*) to 10 (*extreme intensity*) scale. Please complete as many cells as possible, and record activities as close to the time when they actually occurred as you can.

Time	Sunday	Monday	Tuesday	Wednesday	Thursday	Friday	Saturday
12:00 A.M.							
1:00 A.M.							
2:00 A.M.							
3:00 A.M.							
4:00 A.M.							
5:00 A.M.							
6:00 A.M.							
7:00 A.M.							
8:00 A.M.							
9:00 A.M.							
10:00 A.M.							
11:00 A.M.							
12:00 P.M.							
1:00 P.M.							
2:00 P.M.							
3:00 P.M.							
4:00 P.M.							
5:00 P.M.							
6:00 P.M.							
7:00 P.M.							
8:00 P.M.							
9:00 P.M.							
10.00 P.M.							
11:00 P.M.							

FIGURE 4.1. Activity chart.

general activity level, correlations between activity and mood, range of feelings, and ratings of the mastery or pleasure clients derive from their activities. In reviewing activity charts with clients, therapists can also gain a sense of the breadth or restriction of clients' activities. For example, some clients may engage solely in work tasks and have very little relaxation or pleasure, whereas others may show purely passive behaviors, with little accomplishment to feel good about at the end of the day. The former clients may use work as an escape or distraction from feeling blue, whereas the latter may allow necessary tasks of daily life to go undone, increasing feelings of frustration and hopelessness. The activity chart can then be used to guide clients through increasing their activity, to monitor avoidance behaviors, and to evaluate progress toward their life goals.

Activating depressed clients is extremely important. If clients are not engaging in activities that formerly brought them pleasure, or if they are not engaged in important activities that maintain health and well-being, these become a priority in the treatment. The mechanism of change when clients activate is not yet clear. There are several possibilities. The activated client may come in contact with positive reinforcers in his or her natural environment (Jacobson et al., 1996). Getting activated may challenge previously held beliefs about self-efficacy or predictions of negative outcomes as the client engages and discovers that his or her beliefs are not proved to be accurate (Hollon, 2001). Activation may allow clients to develop an understanding of their ability to control many aspects of their lives that they did not recognize because of long-standing hopelessness and helplessness (McCullough, 2001).

Activity scheduling is straightforward. Once the client has gathered baseline data on his or her weekly behaviors on an activity chart, client and therapist begin to look for patterns. Ideally, activity charts include what the client did, who the client was with, and how he or she felt. Situations in which the client recorded that he or she felt better are targeted for increase, whereas situations in which the client stated that he or she felt badly are examined more carefully. The reason that the latter need to be examined rather than simply decreased is that therapists need to be careful not to participate in client avoidance. For example, Rick noted on his activity chart (Figure 4.2) that he felt hopeless on several occasions at work. Avoiding work was a problem behavior to be modified, so he could not simply be encouraged to stay away from work and take more walks in the park (which, he had noted, made him feel "content").

Rick did not complete many of the cells in his activity chart. This is common. Although it would be wonderful if clients completed every piece of homework that therapists provide, they often don't. Homework is given for the client's benefit, not to add further stress. Therapists should point out that clients who complete more of the suggested homework tend to show greater improvements as a result of CBT for depression (Persons, Burns, & Perloff, 1988), but therapists do well to accept and use to optimal benefit any efforts clients make. They can also learn a great deal about a client's behavior and beliefs by examining reasons the client gives for not completing homework. Rick's chart gave his therapist several clues from which to work. Several expressed emo-

Please record the following information in the boxes below: What were you doing? If you were with other people, please note. How were you feeling? Please rate the intensity of the feeling on a 0 (*not at all*) to 10 (*extreme intensity*) scale. Please complete as many cells as possible, and record activities as close to the time when they actually occurred as you can.

Time	Sunday	Monday	Tuesday	Wednesday	Thursday	Friday	Saturday
12:00 A.M.	Watch TV, bored 9	Sleep, unconscious, 10					
1:00 A.M.	Same, bored 10 Tired, 3	,,					
2:00 A.M.	Go to bed, restless, 9	,,					
3:00 A.M.	Computer solitaire, mad, 4	,,					
4:00 A.M.	Finally asleep	,,					
5:00 A.M.	,,	,,					
6:00 A.M.	,,	,,					
7:00 A.M.	,,	,,					
8:00 A.M.	,,	Awake, shower, tired, 10	Awake, tired, 5				
9:00 A.M.	,,	Work, miserable, 8	Walk Sadie, rushed, 9				
10:00 A.M.	,,	,,	Late for work, indifferent, 7				
11:00 A.M.	,,	,,					Awake, coffee, tired, 8
12:00 P.M.	,,	,,					Call from Lou, annoyed, 2
1:00 P.M.	Awake, walk Sadie, guilty, 9	Lunch, Eric, sarcastic, 5					Walk Sadie, guilty, 8
2:00 P.M.	Back to bed, sad, ?	Work, tired miserable, 4					Take Sadie to park, absolved
3:00 P.M.	In bed, lonely, 9	,,					Playing fetch with Sadie, happy, 4
4:00 P.M.	Masturbate, back to bed, sad, 8	,,					
5:00 P.M.	Eat a piece of toast, bored, 9						
6:00 P.M.			Walk Sadie in park, content, 9				
7:00 P.M.							
8:00 P.M.							
9:00 P.M.	Walk Sadie, typical, 8						
10.00 P.M.							
11:00 P.M.			Walk Sadie, nervous, 3				

FIGURE 4.2. Rick's activity chart.

tions needed explaining, such as "typical" on Sunday, "miserable" on Monday, and "guilty" on Saturday and Sunday, when he walked his dog, Sadie.

When Rick's therapist explored the chart with him, it became clear that Rick felt guilty when he overslept and made Sadie wait to be walked. He often awoke from sleep, thought that he should walk the dog, but stayed in bed thinking about what a terrible pet owner he was. When Sadie would whine, he would tell her to go lay down, then roll over, away from her. Rick also felt "miserable" at work, because he spent most of his day checking e-mail and "looking busy." Several projects required his attention, but on the days listed on the activity chart, he spent only a small portion of his workday on them. He recorded that he felt "cynical" when he had lunch with Eric, a coworker, because Eric was very excited about one of the projects and frequently said, "When we get this done, it is going to be very useful." He thought that Eric was a Pollyanna, because he couldn't imagine feeling excited about anything at his job.

After reviewing the activity chart with Rick, his therapist asked him what activities he could agree to engage in more frequently in the next week. One of the things that Rick wanted to do was to awaken earlier on weekend days, so that he could take Sadie out. Because Rick had been sleeping until very late in the afternoon, his therapist suggested a time to awaken that was later than what Rick stated would be ideal but seemed more realistic. Rick also thought that he would turn his television off at 9 P.M. the night before and soak in a hot bath for 20 minutes, one hour prior to going to bed. He and his therapist agreed that Rick would try to be out of bed by 10:00 A.M. on Saturday and Sunday. They also scheduled a small breakfast consisting of a protein bar, coffee, and a piece of fruit. Rick also scheduled a trip to the grocery store for the following Thursday evening to purchase the food items.

Problem Solving

Activating clients requires more than simply scheduling events. It is important to develop a plan for getting goals accomplished (Gollwitzer, 1999) and to rehearse the steps with clients. Therapists need to help clients anticipate obstacles to getting tasks done. Once obstacles are identified, the therapist and client problem-solve to develop a plan for the client to work around the obstacle. The heart of problem solving (D'Zurilla & Nezu, 1982) is to identify the problem and a goal, brainstorm steps toward the goal, choose a plan of action, and review the outcome of the action, modifying the action, if necessary.

During the course of Rick's therapy, increasing social activity was identified as a major goal, as was improving job performance and/or considering alternative employment. These goals required significant problem solving to develop workable plans. Since his partner's death, Rick had become very isolated and was no longer active in the gay community in his city. Like many gay men, he was not interested in going to bars, and he had had significant experience in the bars that taught him that they were a poor venue for making lasting connections with other men. Rick and his therapist developed a list of activities that he could try. His first assignment was to find local gay and lesbian publications, and identify possible social activities from reading the classified section. Asking clients who live in rural or isolated areas to obtain a copy of the national gay yellow pages, or gay and lesbian literature from the nearest urban area, can accomplish the task of finding social groups. The Internet should not be underestimated, either, as a source of ideas for local activities and possible friendships via chat lines or personals. Social connection need not be limited to the LGB communities. However, clients in rural areas can find other activities of interest to them, regardless of whether they are gay events.

Rick obtained a copy of the local gay newspaper and considered all of the activities advertised in the classified section. He discovered, to his surprise, that there were gay hiking groups, bowling teams, bingo nights, churches, and softball leagues in his area. The only group that sounded interesting to him was the hiking group. He could not imagine himself bowling, playing bingo, or attending church. His therapist did not argue with this assessment. They wrote the goal of going on a hike with the hiking group, which met on Saturday mornings at 7 A.M. They then listed the steps that Rick would need to take to make it to the group. The steps included the following:

> Calling the coordinator to find the gathering site.
> Calling the transit authority to inquire about bus routes to the site.
> Finding his hiking boots.
> Buying a water bottle and fanny pack.
> Buying energy bars.
> Checking the weather forecast on the Internet.
> Awakening at 5:30 A.M. on Saturday to allow time to walk Sadie.
> Filling the bottle with chipped ice and cold water.

By far, the greatest obstacle for Rick was to wake early enough to get to the group. He and his therapist planned steps to help him do so. He planned to eat a light meal early in the evening, so that he would not be hungry, because he regularly went without dinner, then awakened in the middle of the night and ate a bowl of cereal. He was then to take

Sadie for a long walk between 7 and 9 P.M. on Friday. When he returned from walking her, he was to change his bedding, because he often slept better on clean sheets. He then was to take a long, warm bath, and drink a glass of warm milk.

Interestingly, as he and his therapist discussed these plans, Rick showed modest excitement about the activity. This is not unusual in some depressed clients as they begin to anticipate positive events more specifically. He was, however, a little afraid of attending the hiking group, because he was uncomfortable meeting new people. He liked to hike, however, and decided that he could enjoy the scenery even if he did not interact very much. His therapist encouraged him to develop a plan for what to say to people. They agreed that Rick would find one or two guys who seemed friendly and ask them how long they had been involved in the hiking group, where they lived, what they did for work, and what other hiking spots they enjoyed. He would also answer any questions that they asked in a forthright manner, even though he did not like talking about his work and worried that people would ask him about that. He agreed to "tell them honestly what I do, but also to redirect the conversation, if I can."

One attempt at an activity is not likely to have a large impact on a client. In the example of Rick's hiking day, he could easily discount any enjoyment as a fluke, so his therapist asked him to commit to attending the group each Saturday for a month prior to making any decisions about whether he thought it was helpful. Rick did join the hiking group on the scheduled Saturday; however, he was more tired than he had hoped, because he had trouble falling asleep, despite the precautions he took. He reported to the therapist that he mostly enjoyed it but that, ultimately, it made him feel more depressed. Three of the men in the group invited him to join them for dinner after they returned from the hike, but he turned them down. The therapist questioned Rick about this:

RICK: The hike was fine, and lots of the guys were friendly. I really thought the guys that asked me to join them for dinner were fun, and that they'd be fun to have dinner with, but . . . (*at this point he stops and his affect turns sad*).

THERAPIST: Something seems to be making you very sad, Rick. You were saying that you thought they'd be fun but . . . what is the "but"?

RICK: Two of them, I think their names were Ron and Gary, looked kind of sick to me. You know, they had that HIV look.

THERAPIST: Can you tell me what you mean?

RICK: They had kind of sunken faces. I noticed that they looked fairly strong in their upper bodies, but that they didn't have any butts, and one of them, Gary, got winded pretty often.

THERAPIST: Did you guys talk about HIV?

RICK: Well, I told them that Anthony had died, and both Gary and Ron had lost several partners. They never told me whether they were sick.

THERAPIST: You thought that they were, however.

RICK: Yes. I just didn't want to get involved.

THERAPIST: I certainly understand that, Rick, but is there anything that you might have missed out on because you didn't want to get involved?

RICK: Yes, I missed out on getting to know them better. Also, the third guy didn't look sick, but who knows? I suppose I could have had a good time with them.

Rick's experience of meeting Ron and Gary had served as a trigger for feeling sad. He made several assumptions about them that were possibly correct but unsubstantiated. He also engaged in his typical avoidance behavior to prevent feeling distressed if they were, in fact, living with HIV. Dealing with client avoidance is important when working with depressed individuals. The alternative to avoidance is approaching situations that may bring distress to move past the distress and obtain positive, long-term gain.

Management of Avoidance

Cognitive-behavioral therapists often use acronyms to assist clients to remember a new plan of action. A short acronym developed to remind clients to break patterns of avoidance is the word "TRAP" (Jacobson, Martell, & Dimidjian, 2001; Martell, Addis, & Jacobson, 2001), representing Trigger, Response, and Avoidance Pattern. Clients are encouraged to get out of the "TRAP" and get back on "TRAC"—that is, the same Trigger and Response but with "AC" standing for Alternative Coping. For Rick, the trigger was seeing men who showed characteristics that he related to HIV disease, the response was to feel sad, and his avoidance pattern was to ruminate about his losses and not interact with the men. The alternative coping was to get to know the men, get accurate information about their health, and enjoy the time spent without planning the entire beginning, middle, and end of the friendship before it had even begun.

As stated earlier, behavioral activation is an integral part of CBT for depression. It can be the predominant method used in the treatment, or it can be used as one intervention in conjunction with other cognitive techniques. Rick's therapy consisted mostly of activation exercises, including his continuing attendance at the hiking group's meetings. He saw Ron at future groups, but Gary did not attend the hiking group for the remainder of the time that Rick attended. He and Ron struck up a friendship, and through Ron, Rick met several other men and women. He continued to have a tendency to isolate himself, but he showed improvement in making contact with these new friends, at least by making an occasional telephone call. Rick also improved his attendance at work and became more involved in the projects that he had previously been avoiding. He recognized that he was generally unhappy in his job; at the time that therapy ended, he was beginning to explore career change options. When Rick completed therapy, his BDI scores were below 10, and his BHS score was a 3, indicating that he was feeling more hopeful. There were still other improvements to be made, but Rick was no longer stuck in the downward spiral of depression and had learned that approaching situations rather than avoiding them helped him to feel better and provided opportunities for enjoyment.

COGNITIVE TECHNIQUES

The ABC theory of emotion proposed first by Ellis (1962) and later by Beck provided an important understanding of the way thoughts can influence mood and behavior for many individuals. In this theory, "A" is an activating event, "B" is a belief, and "C" is a consequence of the belief. Beck et al. (1979) developed a comprehensive treatment for depression that included the behavioral techniques mentioned earlier, as well as cognitive techniques. Caroline's problem list suggested that behavioral activation could help reduce her social isolation and perhaps help her to find employment. However, Caroline also held negative beliefs about herself and negative predictions about the future. Beck et al. (1979) identified a negative triad in depression, consisting of negative views of the self, the world, and the future. Beck recognized that, most of the time, people are not aware of their thinking, and that events are automatically interpreted in negative ways by depressed people. These automatic thoughts (Beck, 1976) are the primary initial targets of cognitive therapy for depression. Clients are taught to identify automatic thoughts; recognize the connection between what they think, and how they feel and behave; examine evidence that supports or contradicts the automatic thought; consider other interpretations of the data; look at the effects of thinking one way versus another; and then to find an alternative response to the thought.

Thought Records

The most convenient tool for working with a client's negative thinking is the Dysfunctional Thought Record (DTR; Beck et al., 1979). There are various forms of thought records, and therapists can purchase packets of cognitive therapy materials or use their own format. Figure 4.3 is an example of a DTR. A variety of formats for thought records exists. Several good texts on cognitive therapy give detailed descriptions of working with clients through a thought record, most notably J. S. Beck (1995) and Greenberger and Padesky (1995). Identifying beliefs and teaching clients to construct alternatives to their dysfunctional thinking is the hallmark of cognitive therapy. During the initial sessions, Caroline was introduced to the ABC theory of emotion. The therapist also helped her to recognize the negative triad in her thinking about herself, her future, and other people. J. S. Beck (1995) and Persons, Davidson, and Tompkins (2001) provide excellent examples of the case formulation with cognitive therapy.

Once Caroline was "on board" with the case formulation and the cognitive model, the therapist asked her to complete the first three columns of a thought record. She was to pay attention to changes in her mood or bodily symptoms (e.g., sighing, tightness in stomach, tearing up) and to note the situation and what went through her mind at the time that her mood shifted. Automatic thoughts may be in the form of ideas or visual images that may flit by quickly but carry important, negative meanings. Many people notice their negative feelings before they notice their thinking, so mood shifts are usually a good cue for clients. Figure 4.4 is one example of the first three columns that Caroline completed for homework.

The situation in which Caroline noticed a shift in her mood to "sad and angry" occurred when her former girlfriend, Charlene, called her and, during the conversation, told her that she had been out on a date with a woman she met while roller-blading. Caroline thought that Charlene was "better off without her" and that she (Caroline) would "never meet a woman and have a happy relationship." She believed both of these thoughts 100%. The fact that she believed them so strongly was an indication of her extreme thinking. It may be possible to believe 100% that one is wearing a blue shirt (if, indeed, one is), but few other things in life allow us such absolute certainty. The situation and the negative thoughts were connected with feelings of sadness and anger.

Situation: Who, what, when, where?	Thought: What were you thinking just before you felt this way (may include visual images)? How much did you believe this (0–100%)?	Feeling: (e.g., sad, angry, scared, happy)	What possible distortions might there be here?		Alternative response: Based on the evidence, what other ways might you view the situation?
			Evidence that supports the thought:	Evidence that does not support the thought:	
					Outcome: How do you feel? Rerate belief in original thought.

FIGURE 4.3. An example of a Dysfunctional Thought Record.

Reviewing Evidence

The theory of cognitive therapy maintains that a person's mood and emotions can be regulated by targeting distortions in thinking and helping clients to interpret situations in a more balanced fashion. One frequent misunderstanding of cognitive therapy, particularly in the treatment of depression, is that clients are expected to think more positively. It must be noted that positive thinking can also be distorted thinking, if there is not evidence to support it. Rather, what cognitive therapists seek is for clients to see things in a more balanced, functional way. Indeed, seeing things in an unrealistically positive manner can pave the way for later, strong disappointment and a rapid drop in mood. Reviewing the evidence for a belief is an important aspect of cognitive therapy for depression. Using the Socratic method (Beck et al., 1979), therapists help clients to evaluate the evidence that supports and does not support their belief, and to construct an alternative response to their original belief. The goal is to have a cognitive shift: decreasing the valence of the dysfunctional belief and increasing the client's accep-

Situation: Who, what, when, where?	Thought: What were you thinking just before you felt this way (may include visual images)? How much did you believe this (0–100%)?	Feeling: (e.g., sad, angry, scared, happy)	What possible distortions might there be here?		Alternative response: Based on the evidence, what other ways might you view the situation?
Tuesday evening, 9:00: Charlene called and told me that she had gone on a date with a woman she met while roller-blading.	*Charlene is better off without me,* 100%. *I'll never meet a woman and have a happy relationship,* 100%.	*Sad* *Angry*	Evidence that supports the thought:	Evidence that does not support the thought:	
					Outcome: How do you feel? Rerate belief in original thought.

FIGURE 4.4. An example of a Thought Record used with Caroline.

tance of a broader perspective. Readers are again referred to J. S. Beck (1995) and Greenberger and Padesky (1995) for excellent descriptions of Socratic questioning and formulating alternative responses to dysfunctional thoughts.

In Caroline's case, the therapist used the thought record to teach her how to construct an alternative response to the thought that Charlene would be better off without her.

THERAPIST: You've done a nice job writing your thoughts and feelings about the telephone call you received from Charlene. It looks like you believed these thoughts very strongly.

CAROLINE: Yes, that's how I saw it.

THERAPIST: Well, today, I'd like to work through the remainder of the thought record with you. If you look at the form, you'll notice that there are columns to write evidence that supports your automatic thought, and evidence that does not support the thought. What do you see as evidence that supports the belief that Charlene is better off without you?

CAROLINE: Well, nobody wants to date a depressed person who can't hold a job.

THERAPIST: Do you think that is evidence for your belief, or is that another belief that you have?

CAROLINE: I don't understand what you mean.

THERAPIST: Well, when you say that nobody wants to date a depressed person, aren't you expressing an idea that you have, in essence, that you believe that nobody wants to do that? Evidence is something more tangible. It would be like telling a judge, "The suspect was really down and out," which would be an opinion, as opposed to saying, "The suspect was wearing ragged jeans, a dirty, torn sweatshirt, and his hair was matted and greasy." Do you see the difference?

CAROLINE: Yes, one is subjective. The other is not.

THERAPIST: Exactly, and I would like you to consider objective evidence, because your thoughts are, by nature, subjective. Can you tell me why that would be helpful?

CAROLINE: To get some objectivity on this problem?

THERAPIST: Exactly. When we look at our thoughts objectively, we can occasionally recognize other possibilities in our interpretations.

CAROLINE: So, then, I guess some objective evidence that my thought is true is that she is now dating someone else.

THERAPIST: Yes, she went on a date with someone else. [Note that the therapist gently corrects Caroline's overgeneralization based on the information Charlene gave her. Charlene had told Caroline that she had gone on a date, and Caroline has turned that into "she is dating" someone. The therapist does not argue with Caroline, or correct her again, after just having tried to explain that Caroline's first attempt at finding evidence was really another belief. Therapists should not appear critical of the client's attempts.]

CAROLINE: Well, also, I don't think that I'll have a relationship, because it didn't work out for Charlene and me, and now that she is not dating me, she has met someone else. So I think that proves both of the thoughts.

THERAPIST: Shall we write those down under evidence that supports the thought [see Figure 4.5]? Is there any other evidence that you can think of that supports your thought?

CAROLINE: Yes, she is the one that went on a date, and I stayed home alone!

THERAPIST: Shall we write that down as well?

CAROLINE: Yes.

THERAPIST: Anything else?

CAROLINE: Not that I can think of.

THERAPIST: Can you think of any evidence that does not support your thinking?

CAROLINE: That is hard to do after finding evidence that clearly supports it. I don't think there is anything. It all seems very clear to me.

THERAPIST: That is the difficult part about this, isn't it? It does all seem very clear. In a minute, we'll talk about the kinds of errors and distortions in thinking that make it so, but I wonder whether, together, we might be able to come up with some evidence that would not support your thoughts.

CAROLINE: I'm willing to try.

THERAPIST: Can you tell me who ended the relationship, you or Charlene?

CAROLINE: I did. I thought she was just going to be brought down by me. I'm such a loser lately . . .

THERAPIST: It seems like there is another belief we will need to deal with, that "you are a loser," but let's try to stay with the thoughts that she is better off without you, and that you won't ever meet a woman and have a happy relationship. So you broke it off. Do you know for a fact that Charlene would not be dating you had you not done that?

CAROLINE: No.

THERAPIST: Is it possible that she would have been happy to have stayed with you and that she understood you are depressed?

CAROLINE: Well, she has made attempts to stay in contact with me, even when I've been rather withdrawn.

THERAPIST: That sounds like evidence that does not support either the belief that she is better off without you or that you won't meet anyone.

CAROLINE: How do you mean?

THERAPIST: Well, you broke off the relationship, but perhaps she would have been happy to stay and is not better off without you; she is just

Situation: Who, what, when, where?	Thought: What were you thinking just before you felt this way (may include visual images)? How much did you believe this (0–100%)?	Feeling: (e.g., sad, angry, scared, happy)	What possible distortions might there be here? *Personalizing* *Overgeneralizing* *Fortune-telling*		Alternative response: Based on the evidence, what other ways might you view the situation?
Tuesday evening, 9:00: Charlene called and told me that she had gone on a date with a woman she met while roller-blading.	*Charlene is better off without me, 100%.* *I'll never meet a woman and have a happy relationship, 100%.*	*Sad* *Angry*	Evidence that supports the thought:	Evidence that does not support the thought:	*Charlene has gone on with her dating life, and still cares enough about me to call me.*
			Now that Charlene is not dating me, she has met someone else. *It didn't work out with Charlene and me.* *She went on a date, and I stayed home alone.*	*I broke off our relationship.* *She wanted to remain friends.* *She only went on one date with this woman.* *I don't go out, so I don't have a chance to meet women.*	Outcome: How do you feel? Rerate belief in original thought. *Still sad, but less so. Not angry.* *She's better off without me, 50%.* *I'll never meet anyone, 70%.*

FIGURE 4.5. An example of a completed Thought Record used with Caroline.

moving forward. Also, you seem to believe that you aren't good enough for a relationship, but she must find something worth pursuing, because she continues the friendship. Shall we write those down?

CAROLINE: Yes, but she may just stay in touch with me because she feels sorry for me.

THERAPIST: There's another belief that calls for evaluation.

CAROLINE: I see that. It's not a fact, is it? I can't get this right.

THERAPIST: You are getting this exactly right. These are the battles we deal with in our minds when we are depressed. It is common to see everything through a negative perspective. So can we take what we have at face value, without trying to guess Charlene's motives, and write that you were the one who broke off the relationship, and that she wanted to remain friends, simply as facts that do not fully support your initial automatic thoughts?

CAROLINE: Yes.

THERAPIST: So, as you look at this, do you still believe that she is better off without you?

CAROLINE: Well, she has only gone on one date with this woman, who could turn out to be an axe murderer for all we know.

THERAPIST: Let's hope not. You know, I just noticed something. Earlier, you said she was dating this woman, and now you've just pointed out that she has only gone on one date. Do you think that is evidence that she may, ultimately, not be better off without you?

CAROLINE: Especially if the woman turns out to be a freak!

THERAPIST: Especially then, but what if she just has gone on one date and has a friend, but nothing really comes of it?

CAROLINE: Yeah, I guess we can include that, but she goes out a lot and will always meet someone.

THERAPIST: And what about you?

CAROLINE: What do you mean, "What about me?"

THERAPIST: Do you go out?

CAROLINE: You know I don't.

THERAPIST: Yes, I know that, and if you don't go out, how do you know whether you'll ever meet someone?

CAROLINE: Well, if I don't go out, I won't have the chance to meet anyone.

THERAPIST: Yes, but if you did go out, you might have the chance. So shall we write that because you don't go out, you don't have the chance to meet other women, as evidence that doesn't support the belief that you'll never meet another woman? "Never" is a very strong word, especially since you don't know what would happen if you did start going out again.

CAROLINE: Yes, sure.

THERAPIST: I'd like you to take a look at this evidence we've gathered, and then take a look again at the original automatic thoughts. Can you identify any possible errors in logic that you made initially?

CAROLINE: Well, it seems that I made it all about me when she told me that she had gone on a date. Also, I had her basically married to this woman in my mind, when she had only gone on one date.

THERAPIST: So we can call that personalizing, because when we make things about us when they may not be, we are either making ourselves responsible or implying that others have motives for their behavior that have to do with us in some way even, when they may not. Marrying her off after a first date we would call overgeneralizing, right?

CAROLINE: Yes, I can see that. I think I'm also trying to predict the future.

THERAPIST: How so?

CAROLINE: By saying I'll never meet anyone.

THERAPIST: Yes, I see that. Shall we write these three things—personalizing, overgeneralizing, and predicting the future or fortunetelling—here in the box that identifies distortions in thinking?

CAROLINE: Yes.

THERAPIST: So, given the evidence that supports and does not support the automatic thought, can you think of an alternative response that is not personalized, overgeneralized, or fortune-telling?

CAROLINE: Well, I guess she's gone on with her life but still wants me in it.

THERAPIST: Yes, that is true, but I wonder, is there something specific that she has gone on with?

CAROLINE: Her dating life.

THERAPIST: Do you see how that is even less overgeneralized?

CAROLINE: Yes, so let's say that "Charlene has gone on with her dating life, and still cares enough to call me." I think that would be true.

THERAPIST: I think that is excellent. Now, when you think about it that way, how do you feel?

CAROLINE: I still feel sad, but not as much. I don't feel angry anymore, because I don't feel dumped.

THERAPIST: Let's write that down under the outcome. You also believed the automatic thoughts 100% initially. Do you still believe them that strongly?

CAROLINE: No, I think I believe that she is better off without me about 50%, because I don't know what will happen to her. I still believe that I'm unlikely to meet anyone or have a happy relationship, because I don't know whether I'll ever get over this depression.

THERAPIST: How strongly do you believe that, still 100%?

CAROLINE: No, about 70%, I guess.

THERAPIST: So as we've gone through this thought record, you've had a slight shift in your feelings. You are less sad and not angry, and you believe your initial thoughts a little less strongly. You've been able to find an alternative interpretation of the situation when Charlene called you that is a little more balanced, and that does not make it about you, overgeneralize, or predict the future. Can you tell me your reaction to this method? [The therapist has summarized the activity for Caroline and is now eliciting feedback. Frequent summaries and gathering feedback are essential components in CBT, because they ensure that the client understands the point of the discussion and maintains the spirit of collaboration.]

CAROLINE: Well, I don't think that I can be this logical, especially when I'm really down.

THERAPIST: I understand that it is difficult when you're down. Do you think it is worth trying?

CAROLINE: What if I said "no"?

THERAPIST: Well, we'd need to figure something else out.

CAROLINE: I guess, actually, it would be good to try. I used to like to be logical, and I've been that way in school before.

THERAPIST: So this is a way to apply logical analysis when you are feeling badly about a particular situation. It may not always make you feel better, but often it may. The more you do this, the easier it will get. I'll ask you to use the written thought record to do the analysis, because we are trying to help you develop a new habit. The more concrete we can be, the better, when trying to break the old habitual way of depressive thinking and to develop a new habit of finding balanced alternatives.

A client can be taught to ask him- or herself many questions that will help in finding alternative responses to automatic thoughts. The most frequent question is "What evidence is there that the thought is true?" Any question that assists the client to recognize distortions in thinking and to get emotional distance from the thought is a valid question.[1]

Old Belief/New Belief

Some client beliefs are prevalent across situations in their lives. They are stereotypical ways of interpreting situations that clients have learned in many situations, and frequently are absolute statements about themselves or the world. Caroline's feeling that she is a "loser" is such a belief. Some people make statements about themselves, such as "I'm a loser," but do not really believe them. Others don't necessarily verbalize such thoughts but live their lives and make other choices as if it were true that they are indeed losers.

Once clients have become proficient at using thought records, they can expand the method to tackle these core beliefs. Once such method for dealing with core beliefs is the "old belief/new belief" technique (J. S. Beck, 1995; Persons, 1989). Clients state their old belief. Then, they write evidence that supports and does not support that belief. In some cases, it is good to ask them to write a reframe of the evidence that allegedly supports the old belief (J. S. Beck, 1995). For example, Caroline said that losing her first job out of college proved that she was a loser. The reframe for this piece of evidence was that she had been targeted by an unjust supervisor and might not have lost her job because of her performance. The client is then asked to state a new belief that, to some extent, contradicts the old one. Caroline stated the new belief, "I am a capable young woman." Note that she did not say, "I am a winner." Therapists must take care to help clients refrain from such dichotomies. They are usually not true, and they are often not believable. A person cannot describe him- or herself as a winner, because there are surely times when one loses. It is as distorted as saying "I am a loser." The belief, "I am a capable young woman," is more balanced and lends itself to affirmative evidence. The client then lists evidence that supports the new belief. Clients can also rate the degree to which they believe the old belief, then develop the new belief, and, at the end of the exercise, rerate the strength of their old belief.

COMBINING COGNITIVE AND BEHAVIORAL ELEMENTS

In most instances of CBT for depression, the therapist makes use of both behavioral and cognitive elements. Clients can be given assignments to conduct behavioral experiments to test their beliefs. Caroline, for example, was given the assignment of going out to a local garden shop where many single, lesbian women were known to shop, and simply to smile and say "hello" as she passed. This was to test her belief, "Nobody pays attention to me." Her therapist helped her to formulate an alternative belief, "People will notice me if I engage in simple social discourse." The latter idea was actively tested by the assignment to say "hello" to women she passed in the garden center. It was not necessary to engage in conversation, to collect phone numbers, or engage in any other threatening behavior. Caroline simply needed to collect data on how many women responded in some way to her, either negatively or positively. She discovered, to her surprise, that 99% of the women to whom she said "hello" smiled and said hello back. The one woman who did not was carrying a rose bush to the counter, and scratched herself with a thorn seconds after she made eye contact with Caroline, so Caroline considered that the woman was preoccupied, and didn't take it personally. Although her experiment did not produce earth-shattering findings, this simple assignment allowed Caroline to see that her belief could not be absolutely true; if so many women responded to her greeting, she could not have gone unnoticed.

Behavioral components of CBT can not only be used simply to activate a lethargic, withdrawn, or passive depressed individual, but also to test beliefs, as in the previous example. The cognitive components are used to teach clients to look at the world in a less stereotypically negative way. CBT for depression is active, and therapists need to encourage clients to complete homework tasks and to actively collaborate in the sessions. Therapists should take care not to do all the work for the client, however, because depressed clients frequently evoke this response from their therapists (McCullough, 2001).

LGB individuals often have to replace old beliefs about themselves with new beliefs. The majority of LGB people are raised to believe that they will develop into heterosexual adults, and that it is abnormal or even bad not to do so. The first belief that is challenged during the coming-out process is that it is abnormal to be LGB. Most LGB people successfully develop new beliefs about themselves and the worlds in which they live, without developing psychiatric conditions such as depression. However, when working with a depressed LGB client, it is good to assess the client's belief about him- or herself. As discussed in Chapter 1, LGB individuals may believe the negative ideas and stereotypes about homosexuality, and maintain dysfunctional attitudes and expectations for their lives. When LGB adults are depressed and seek therapy, CBT is a powerful tool for helping them to engage fully in their lives and to appreciate themselves as healthy people who can contribute much to society and have loving relationships and meaningful lives.

Chapter 5

Anxiety Disorders

Erik: Social Anxiety Disorder

Erik, a 35-year-old, gay, white male, presented for treatment after seeing a television commercial about medications for social anxiety disorder. He was not interested in psychotropic medications. However, this advertisement drew his attention to the fact that he might suffer from social anxiety. Since the time he graduated from college, Erik had been working as a paralegal in a law firm. Because of his anxiety about attending law school and becoming a lawyer himself, and about interviewing for jobs, he had remained in the same job for years. He felt that he was "comfortable enough" at his current job, and this feeling exacerbated his fear-related avoidance. For example, over time, his coworkers had come to know about his sexual orientation, and he felt comfortable with them having this knowledge. To avoid having either to "come out" at a new position or school situation or to dodge personal questions in a new work environment, he had slowly and gradually forsaken many of his career-related goals. He had started working at this firm right after college, thinking it would be a temporary position. He gradually received promotions and raises, and despite his desire to move upward for employment or schooling, he had not made a move in 14 years.

Erik also feared situations that involved meeting new people socially. He avoided social activities such as going on dates and attending functions with other gay men. Although he wanted to be in a significant relationship with another man, he did not put himself in situations where he would meet prospective partners. His main sexual outlet came from one- or two-time encounters with partners he would meet on the Internet. Occasionally, some of these partners would want to continue a relationship with him, but Erik would never return their calls, interpreting their persistence as "They are just being nice" and "If they got to know me better, they would not like me." Additionally, in sexual situations, because of his social anxiety, Erik would sometimes fear being assertive; therefore, he would not discuss or initiate condom use if his partner did not do so. Although luckily he had remained HIV negative, he did contract HPV (genital warts), which further contributed to his avoidance of meeting prospective, long-term partners. He feared that if he were to meet someone, he would eventually have to tell him about this; Erik was mortified by the prospect.

Unsurprisingly, most of Erik's friends were women—some were also paralegals at his office, and others that he had known from college. He felt less anxious around women, because he thought they would be more accepting of his sexual orientation. With women, he also did not fear being romantically rejected. He lived by himself in an apartment, in a medium-size metropolitan city, and spent about half of his weekends alone. During these times, his anxiety would sometimes lead to depressed mood and hopelessness; however, he did not have such feelings during the week when he would go to work and have social contacts.

Erik reported that he had been suffering from social anxiety for quite some time. He believed that this began when he was in junior high school, when he began to feel different from other boys his age. Although he did well in his classes throughout high school, he had a difficult time with his peers and only had a few friends. During this time, Erik began to realize that he had sexual and emotional attractions toward some of the other male adolescents in his class. Erik also did not excel in "male" team sports such as soccer, baseball, or football; this, he felt, also reduced his ability to make friends. As required by his school, he did participate in some athletics and did well with more solitary sports such as long-distance running.

Erik felt that he had always had anxiety throughout his life. He recalled that, even in elementary school, he was shy. He would frequently excuse himself from lunch or recess, complaining of spurious stomach distress. Frequently, he would be unable to eat in front of others in the school cafeteria. His parents were very concerned with appearances. He recalled that manners were extremely important to his mother, and that his parents' behaviors were most extreme when they would have company or go to one of their friends' homes. In such situations, they required that he remained quiet, "shushed" him if he joined conversations, and became excessively angry with him (punishing him by yelling or "grounding him") if his behavior in front of others was contrary to what they wanted. Notably, he also experienced harsh responses from his parents if he engaged in behavior that was in some way considered to be gender-atypical (i.e., wanting to play games such as "house," or play with stuffed animals).

ANNA: GENERALIZED ANXIETY DISORDER

Anna, a 25-year-old, self-identified lesbian woman, presented for treatment of anxiety. At the time of treatment, Anna was in the middle of her first semester of her second year of working toward her social work degree. She had two "incompletes" from her first year, mainly consequences of her excessive worry. Anna was intelligent and appeared to have the skills necessary to be a great social worker. However, she perceived that her worrying was out of control. She reported that she worried during almost all of her waking hours, and reported that the only time she got relief from her worry was when she drank alcohol; however, she did not do this to excess, because she knew she needed to develop alternate ways of handling her worry.

Anna came from a strict family, and her parents placed strong emphasis on educational excellence. If, for example, she returned from school with anything less than an A- or B+ during high school, her parents would restrict her free time and monitor her work—even during her senior year. This did not occur during college, because Anna lived at school, but at this time, she became more and more concerned with perfectionism. She would worry about her schoolwork so excessively that she would not be able to concentrate on it. As a result, she would typically wait until the last minute to finish anything. Thanks to her high intelligence, she completed college successfully with a grade point average (GPA) in the somewhat above-average range.

During college, however, she began to realize that she had attractions for other women. Given her family's traditional views on gender roles and her fears of their reactions, Anna suppressed these feelings. She gradually fell in love with Sarah, her best friend, who returned her affections. At the time of treatment, the two were living together but had two bedrooms in their apartment, so that when family members came to visit, they would not be offended. She had, however, previously discussed her sexual orientation with them, and her father, particularly, did not approve. In fact, for the first 3 months after she told them, he told Anna that he no longer wanted to have contact with her. However, with Anna's mother's help, her father slowly began to see her again but would not talk about the sexual orientation issue.

At the time of treatment, the relationship with her girlfriend was suffering because Anna was so worried about schoolwork, she would avoid engaging in any outside activities and spending time with her. However, when she sat down to do schoolwork, she would become so anxious about getting all of the material correct that she would end up procrastinating. She used the Internet, cleaned the house, or just stared at the computer screen, worrying about her ability ever to complete the amount of required reading. Furthermore, because her program required a lot of challenging reading, her worry was such that she had difficulty concentrating on the material, and would have to reread it several times to get any of it.

Anna's anxiety was exacerbated by her family situation. Despite their discussions with her about her sexual orientation, her parents continually asked her when she would find a boyfriend and get married. This pressure, she believed, contributed to her general pressure to achieve in school, as well as, generally, to be a "perfect" person in every way. Her partner, Sarah, complained that Anna had become more and more irritable, and that they had stopped doing anything fun together because Anna worried about schoolwork "constantly." In fact, many arguments ensued, because it seemed to Sarah that all Anna wanted to talk about was her worries. It felt to Sarah that the majority of their interactions involved Anna verbalizing worries and Sarah trying to help her with these worries.

OVERVIEW OF THE ANXIETY DISORDERS FROM A COGNITIVE-BEHAVIORAL PERSPECTIVE

The core feature of anxiety disorders is perceived threat or danger. Although most people sometimes suffer from fear or anxiety, an individual who suffers from an anxiety disorder has excessive fear, to the point that it causes significant distress and interferes in his or her life. Furthermore, to be considered an anxiety disorder, the fear must be persistent and significantly impair at least one area of role function, such as school, work, one's social life, or relationships. The most recent epidemiological survey estimated that 17.2% of individuals in the United States suffer from an anxiety disorder using a 12-month prevalence estimation, and that 24.95% have a lifetime history of any anxiety disorder (Kessler et al., 1994). These estimations, however, do not include posttraumatic stress disorder.

There are five main anxiety disorders according to the fourth edition of the *Diagnostic and Statistical Manual of Mental Disorders* (DSM-IV; American Psychiatric Association, 1994): social phobia (or social anxiety disorder (SAD), generalized anxiety disorder (GAD), posttraumatic stress disorder (PTSD), panic disorder (PD), obsessive–compulsive disorder (OCD), and specific phobias. We emphasize SAD and GAD in this chapter, and PTSD in Chapter 7. One's sexual orientation is typically not a significant part of CBT for panic disorder or simple phobias;

therefore, treatment of these two anxiety disorders is not emphasized in this book. The case examples in this chapter show how sexual orientation does play a role in treatment for SAD and GAD, even though the general tenets of a validated cognitive-behavioral treatment remain the same regardless of the client's sexual orientation.

The core feature of SAD is a marked fear of embarrassment or humiliation in the presence of others. This can take the form of a specific fear, such as fear of public speaking, or a more generalized set of fears that might include meeting new people, interacting with others, maintaining or initiating conversations, or eating and drinking in public. The central component of GAD is excessive worry about a number of events or activities in one's life, typically accompanied by somatic symptoms of anxiety, such as sleep problems, tension, restlessness, and others. Most theories of the development of anxiety disorders follow a diathesis–stress model; therefore, both biological and environmental factors play a role (see Barlow, 1988, 2001a). Evidence for the biological contribution comes from research on families, twins, and sibling studies. One line of research revealed a dispositional trait—"behavioral inhibition" (see Kagan, 1994). This trait (characterized by shyness and timidity) is present in young childhood, and children with behavioral inhibition are more likely to go on to develop anxiety disorders during midchildhood, adolescence, or adulthood. Family and twin studies also reveal a biological component to the development of anxiety disorders. However, these studies, like studies of most psychiatric disorders, reveal that environmental factors also play a major role.

Untreated anxiety disorders can run a chronic and unremitting course, but empirically validated treatments exist for these problems (see Barlow, 2001a). For each of the anxiety disorders, structured cognitive-behavioral treatments can reduce the degree of anxiety— showing efficacy similar to that of medications (see Barlow, 2001b; Pollack, Otto, & Rosenbaum, 1996). Furthermore, cognitive-behavioral treatments for anxiety disorders lead to improvements in functional impairment and quality of life (e.g., Eng, Coles, Heimberg, & Safren, 2001; Safren, Heimberg, Brown, & Holle, 1997), and some emerging evidence indicates that once the treatment is discontinued, treatment gains are maintained to an even greater degree than those made with psychopharmacology (see Pollack et al., 1996).

LGB People Aren't the Only Anxious Ones

Comparative studies of the prevalence of anxiety disorders in LGB populations are emerging but are generally limited by sample sizes, volunteer samples, or brief screenings (see Gilman et al., 2001). Some studies may have overestimated the prevalence of mental health issues by using biased samples (see Gonsiorek, 1996). Recent population-based studies with unbiased sampling generally estimate that rates of anxiety disorders in LGB populations are similar or greater than those in general samples. Gilman et al. (2001), using data from the National Comorbidity Study (NCS) found that women with same-sex partners had higher 12-month prevalence rates of PTSD and simple phobias than women with same-sex partners, and that men with same-sex partners were significantly more likely to suffer from any anxiety disorder than those with no same-sex partners. The rates of other disorders in this study were similar. Cochran and Mays (2000), using the National Household Survey of Drug Abuse, found that homosexually active men were more likely to experience PD than heterosexual men. These studies are, however, limited because the samples of LGB individuals were quite low. However, anxiety disorders are quite prevalent in general populations, and if the rates are similar in LGB populations, clinicians who treat LGB individuals are bound to confront patients with anxiety disorders.

Two emerging studies report on sexual minority patients. These two studies have come from the mental health department of Fenway Community Health, a community health center that serves large numbers of LGB individuals. Rogers, Emanuel, and Bradford (2003) found that of the women who presented at the mental health department, high percentages had clinically significant anxiety symptoms as rated by their clinician. Mimiaga, Burg, and Safren (2002), in a similar chart review study of the men (who report that they have sex with other men) at Fenway, also found high rates of clinician-reported anxiety symptoms among these men presenting for treatment. The Netherlands Mental Health Survey and Incidence Study (NEMESIS), an epidemiological study, compared homosexually active women and men with heterosexually active women and men (Sandfort, de Graaf, Bijl, & Schnabel, 2001). Men and women with same-sex sexual partners evidenced more mood and anxiety disorders than those with opposite-sex sexual partners.

From a theoretical and developmental point of view, anxiety can become a significant factor for any stigmatized group. From a developmental or social-learning perspective (which are both consistent with cognitive-behavioral models), it makes sense that adolescents who are more likely to face discrimination, harassment, rejection, or even verbal or physical abuse as a result of their sexual orientation (see Savin-Williams, 1994; Savin-Williams & Cohen, 1996) would go on to develop mood or anxiety disorders. Social anxiety can be a barrier to social support (Safren & Pantalone, in press) that could otherwise buffer the effects of stress (e.g., Cohen & Wills, 1985; Sarason, Sarason, &

Pierce, 1990). General anxiety also can occur as an overgeneralization of realistic fears of rejection when developing one's sexual minority identity (see Patterson, 1995; Rotheram-Borus & Fernandez, 1995).

The Three-Component Model as a Basis for Both Assessment and Treatment

In general, the conceptualization and treatment of anxiety disorders from a cognitive-behavioral perspective focuses on a three-component model of anxiety (Figure 5.1). These components (discussed earlier)—cognitive, behavioral, and physiological—are widely accepted in theoretical works about anxiety disorders (e.g., Barlow, 2001a) and serve as the basis for treatment in anxiety disorder treatment manuals (e.g., Barlow, 2001b; Hope, Heimberg, Juster, & Turk, 2000; Rothbaum & Foa, 2000; Zinbarg, Craske, Barlow, & O'Leary, 1993). However, these models are somewhat simplified for treatment, and other, more complex models of the development and maintenance of anxiety disorders exist (see Barlow, 2001a; Menin, Turk, & Heimberg, 2003; Otto & Safren, 2000; Rapee & Heimberg, 1997).

The cognitive component refers to one's thoughts, beliefs, and perceptions about the excessively feared situation or phobic object. For example, Erik (described earlier) has fears about job interviews. When he envisioned going on an interview, he had thoughts such as "I won't know the right thing to say" or "The interviewer will be able to tell I am gay, and he won't like me." In CBT, we consider negative, phobic-related thoughts "automatic," because they happen quickly, without full evaluation, and are likely based on one's learning history and even questioned by the person in the situation.

The main behavioral component of anxiety is avoidance. The acts of avoiding the target of one's anxiety and having negative thoughts about the target of one's anxiety reinforce each other. For example, the negative automatic thoughts and beliefs might be predictions that exposure to the target of one's anxiety will lead to a bad outcome. By avoiding the anxiety-provoking situation, an anxious person can maintain his or her beliefs about the dangerousness of the target. In Erik's case, he completely avoided job interviews, dating, or any situation in which he would meet other gay men as friends or potential relationships. Therefore, Erik could never learn whether the feared situation was actually dangerous, and could never gain skills in learning how to cope with existing anxiety in these situations.

The physiological component of anxiety includes somatic symptoms—the "fight-or-flight" response—and is thought to have an evolutionary basis (see Barlow, 2001a). Symptoms can include sweating, rapid heart-

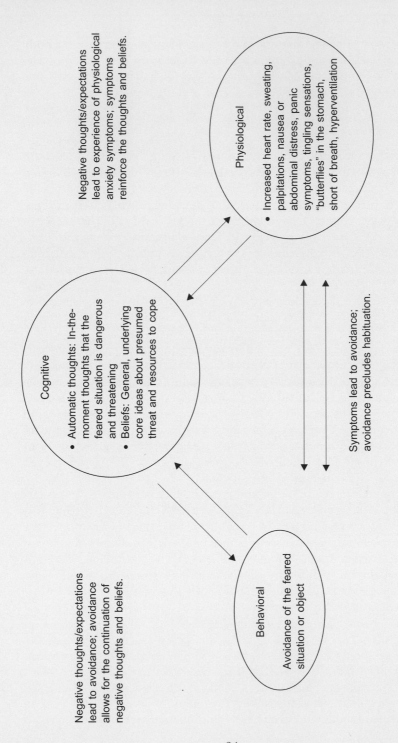

FIGURE 5.1. Three-component model of anxiety.

Negative thoughts/expectations lead to experience of physiological anxiety symptoms; symptoms reinforce the thoughts and beliefs.

Physiological

• Increased heart rate, sweating, palpitations, nausea or abdominal distress, panic symptoms, tingling sensations, "butterflies" in the stomach, short of breath, hyperventilation

Cognitive

• Automatic thoughts: In-the-moment thoughts that the feared situation is dangerous and threatening
• Beliefs: General, underlying core ideas about presumed threat and resources to cope

Symptoms lead to avoidance; avoidance precludes habituation.

Negative thoughts/expectations lead to avoidance; avoidance allows for the continuation of negative thoughts and beliefs.

Behavioral

Avoidance of the feared situation or object

beat, shaking, stomach distress, and others. They help prepare the body to cope with a threatening situation, such as fighting an attacker or fleeing from something dangerous. The response to having such symptoms (which many people experience as aversive or distressing) can reinforce the behavioral component of anxiety: To avoid having symptoms, a person avoids the situations that cause them. They can also add to the cognitive component of anxiety: One can interpret these physiological responses as supporting the emotional reasoning that because they are afraid, the situation must be dangerous. In the case of social phobia, the physiological symptoms can add to a person's fear that other people may notice his or her anxiety and be hostile, judgmental, and unsympathetic.

Structured interviews or assessment instruments such as the Anxiety Disorders Interview Schedule for DSM-IV (ADIS-IV; DiNardo et al., 1994) and the Structured Clinical Interview for DSM-IV (SCID-IV; First et al., 1997), can assist a clinician in differentiating an anxiety disorder from "normal" anxiety. Self-report measures of anxiety can indicate whether someone is likely to be in the clinical range for a disorder. These measures also can be used throughout treatment to monitor progress and continually guide the direction of the treatment. In general, these measures have applicability to LGB populations. However, minor modifications may make these more user-friendly to sexual minority patients. The next sections of this chapter focus on two examples of anxiety disorders: social phobia and GAD. By using the model of the cognitive, behavioral, and physiological components as a basis for both assessment and treatment, more specific information is given, with an example case for both of these anxiety disorders.

SOCIAL ANXIETY DISORDER

Cognitive-Behavioral Assessment

The case of Erik was introduced earlier. After the general assessment and diagnosis of SAD, the therapist began by establishing a baseline level of anxiety and avoidance. First, Erik and his therapist collaboratively completed the Leibowitz Social Anxiety Scale (see Heimberg et al., 1999; Safren et al., 1999). This scale presents a list of 24 social situations and involves rating each item for anxiety (0–3, denoting *none*, *mild*, *moderate*, or *severe anxiety*) and for avoidance (0–3, denoting *never*, *occasionally*, *often*, and *usually*). This clinician-rated form complemented self-report measures, in that the therapist was able to clarify what Erik meant when classifying a symptom with words such as "mild" versus "moderate." The use of this assessment revealed that Erik would avoid many situations in which he felt anxious. Specifically, it showed higher ratings in situations such as "going to a party," "meeting strangers," and "looking at people you do not know very well in the eye." Due to the extensive time involved in completing the assessment, the therapist used this scale only three times: at the start of treatment, midway through, and at the end.

For a less time-consuming assessment, Erik completed the social interaction anxiety scale (see Brown et al., 1997; Mattick & Clarke, 1998; Safren, Heimberg, & Turk, 1998) with the item that asks about "attractive members of the opposite sex" changed to "people I am attracted to." Erik completed this scale in the waiting room before each appointment. His baseline score was also in the range indicative of marked social interaction anxiety (Heimberg, Mueller, Holt, Hope, & Liebowitz, 1992). These two measures, the Leibowitz Social Anxiety Scale, and the Social Interaction Anxiety Scale, were primarily used to monitor progress throughout the treatment and to determine whether the treatment targets were focusing adequately on Erik's areas of interfering anxiety.

Erik and his therapist also developed a fear hierarchy as the base for anxiety "exposures." Cognitive-behavioral therapists use fear hierarchies in the assessment and treatment of most anxiety disorders, and, in the case of SAD, the fear hierarchy is a list of social situations that the patient fears or avoids. In creating the fear hierarchy, the idea is to come up with a list of social situations of varying levels of feared intensity that the patient can then progressively practice. Role-played and imaginative practice can occur in session, as well as *in vivo* practice outside of sessions. The latter is essential for transfer and maintenance of therapeutic gains. For each item, Erik rated how much he feared the situation on a scale of 1–100, and how much he avoided the item on a similar scale. Ideally (as illustrated in Figure 5.2), a fear hierarchy should have items at both ends of the fear spectrum: From items that the patient does fear and avoid but can envision himself doing, or that he sometimes does but endures with anxiety (items ranging from about 20 to 40 on the 1–100 scale), to more moderate fears (items ranging from 40 to 70) and more intense, severe fears (ranging from 70 to 100). This list becomes the base for structuring graded exposure sessions.

When developing a fear hierarchy, Erik and his therapist noted several themes, and each was discussed. First, the overwhelming majority of the fears centered on his personal life and other gay men, rather than on his work situation. Second, they learned situations were dramatically different depending on who else was present in them. Third, as is true of most fear hierarchies, the anxiety rating was similar to the avoidance rating but not identical. For example, Erik rated non-bar gay-oriented

Situation	Anxiety rating	Avoidance rating
1. Being assertive with a female coworker (e.g., saying "no" to an unreasonable request, or requesting something reasonable but that would require extra work for her).	20	30
2. Going out to eat at a gay restaurant with a female friend.	30	40
3. Going to a gay bar, only talking if someone else initiates the conversation.	40	40
4. Returning an item or being assertive with a waiter at a restaurant, where one thinks the waiter is gay.	45	80
5. Being assertive with a male coworker (e.g., saying "no" to an unreasonable request, or requesting something reasonable but that would require more work for him).	45	65
6. Having an in-person conversation with a gay man to whom one has been introduced to by a mutual friend at a social event (where other people are present).	55	10
7. Going to a non-bar gay-oriented event (e.g., such as a gay church event or gay hiking club), only talking if someone else initiates the conversation.	65	100
8. Going on a blind date (nonsexual) with someone one has met on the Internet or through a friend.	70	50
9. Going to a party where one knows some gay people will be.	75	10
10. Initiating a conversation with an attractive gay man.	85	99
11. Going on a job or school interview.	90	100
12. Going to a non-bar gay-oriented event (e.g., gay church or gay hiking club) and initiating a conversation with someone there.	95	100
13. Going to a gay bar and initiating a conversation with a new person.	100	100

FIGURE 5.2. Fear hierarchy for Erik (social anxiety disorder).

events only a 65 for anxiety (number 7), but he had never attended one of these events; therefore, he had to rate the avoidance as 100. This type of situation would therefore be a good intermediate or beginning goal of the treatment. Because of the preponderance of situations involving his social life with other gay men, Erik decided he would like this to be the primary focus of treatment, and that, after these goals were met, he and his therapist would reevaluate the job-related fears.

Moving from Assessment to Treatment

After the diagnostic assessment, the first several sessions of CBT for SAD typically include providing psychoeducational information about social anxiety and its treatment. This is done to establish the credibility of treatment and the client's confidence in it, because greater credibility and confidence in SAD treatment is associated with greater outcome (see Safren, Heimberg, & Juster, 1997). In general, anxiety disorder treatment involves the patient doing the exact thing that has caused him or her the most distress, so to get the client to agree to such a thing, he or she must understand and believe the rationale. Erik and his therapist discussed the simplified three-component model of SAD (cognitive, behavioral, and physiological), with emphasis on each component individually, as well as how each component influences the others, causing a cycle of continued excessive anxiety.

Erik and his therapist first discussed the cognitive component of anxiety, using an example that had come up during the assessment: A coworker, Mary, wanted to introduce him to a friend of hers.

THERAPIST: OK, so what I want you to do is picture yourself thinking about being introduced to this guy. You are at Mary's house. There are several other men and women there, and Mary says to you, "Hey, let me introduce you now." What thoughts immediately come to mind? What do you picture happening?

ERIK: Oh, my God, I'd be so anxious!

THERAPIST: OK, so that is what you will be *feeling*, a rush of anxiety. What will be *going through your head*, making you feel anxious?

ERIK: All I can think of is that he won't want to talk to me.

THERAPIST: Let me write that down. What else might go through your head?

ERIK: I won't have anything to say, and if I do, I'll be so nervous that he will be able to tell that I am anxious.

THERAPIST: OK, I see. Now let's say you do go there, and you do start to talk to him, what would be the worst thing about appearing nervous, or having him noticing that you are anxious?

ERIK: Well, if I look nervous, he won't like me. He will think I am attracted to him, and he will think I am a loser. Basically, he will see my anxiety and reject me.

THERAPIST: So, in your mind, looking nervous means being a loser.

ERIK: Yes. The other thing that goes through my head in these situations is how pathetic I am. I mean, it's just ridiculous that I can't even talk to people because of anxiousness. It makes me think that if even talking to someone is hard for me, I will never be able to meet anyone, and never have a relationship.

THERAPIST: I see. Let me ask you one more question. Let's say you begin to talk with him, and the two of you don't hit it off. What would that mean to you in this situation?

ERIK: It just makes me think that no one would ever like me, and that I will never have a relationship, ever. I might as well give up.

Erik had many negative automatic thoughts about this situation, and beliefs that extended beyond it, including prediction of a negative outcome. Not only did Erik's thoughts stay specifically on this situation but they also triggered beliefs that were internal to him (e.g., "How pathetic *I am*"), global (e.g., "I can't talk to *people*" vs. this specific person), and stable (e.g., "I will *never* be able to meet anyone") (see Seligman, 1998). Anxious and depressed clients frequently have a negative bias about both negative events, as just illustrated, and positive events in the opposite direction: external (e.g., "The instructor was easy on me"); specific (e.g., "I was lucky because I understand simple math") and unstable (e.g., "Tests are usually not this easy"). This negative bias further impedes their interpretations of positive events that could weaken the basis for such schemas.

The behavioral component can be seen as a direct consequence of these negative thoughts and beliefs. Anxious individuals are hypervigilant to external events and interoceptive cues that they interpret as threatening. The main behavioral component for Erik (and with most individuals with SAD) was avoiding the situations that made him anxious. The therapist and Erik then discussed the physiological component of social anxiety for Erik. In feared social situations, Erik would typically experience symptoms such as sweating, increased heart rate, and tingling sensations in his stomach. These would exacerbate his fears, because he felt that his anxiety would be noticeable to and negatively viewed by others; therefore, his anxiety about showing physiological symptoms in social situations would, in turn, cause further anxiety. After a discussion and elicitation of these fears, the therapist added to the cognitive components thoughts and beliefs such as "People will notice my anxiety symptoms" and "If people see that I am anxious, they will think that I am a loser."

Erik's therapist pointed out how each component of anxiety reinforces the other two:

THERAPIST: So let's review where we stand.

ERIK: OK.

THERAPIST: First, we talked about these negative thoughts (*pointing to the three-circle model*, Figure 5.3). If a person is thinking, "I won't

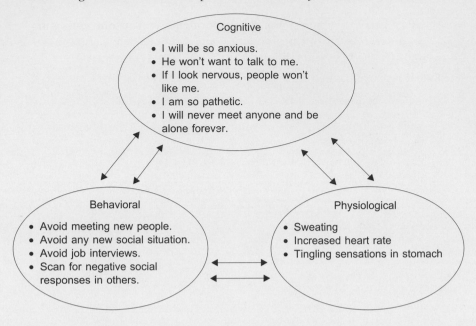

FIGURE 5.3. Erik's thoughts, behaviors, and physical symptoms.

have anything to say" or "He will reject me," what are the chances that he is going to approach someone?

ERIK: Well, pretty slim, I guess.

THERAPIST: Right, these are pretty strong thoughts. So I can really see that if you think these thoughts, you are more likely to avoid approaching someone. So I am going to draw an arrow here, from the cognitive circle to the behavioral circle. Now, when you do avoid, does a person get a chance to learn about the situation or test out whether the thoughts are true or not?

ERIK: I know that they are true.

THERAPIST: I see what you are saying. I understand that these are valid thoughts that you are having. I am just asking, in general, do you think that if a person avoids a situation that he fears, he would get a chance to learn whether his fears are true?

ERIK: Well, not really.

THERAPIST: OK, so I am going to draw an arrow back from the behavioral to the cognitive component. Emphasizing that it's a cycle. Now, let's turn to the physiological component. If someone is having these anxiety-provoking thoughts, and believes that a situation is dangerous, he is probably going to have symptoms.

ERIK: I suppose.

THERAPIST: So there is a link between the cognitive component and the physiological component.

This dialogue continued emphasizing how each component of anxiety reinforces the others. The therapist, then explained that, given this pattern, they would use skills in CBT training not only to attack directly each component of anxiety but also to try to break these connections. Hence, even if a person has anxiety symptoms, it is still important to get through the situation so that one can practice it, habituate to the anxiety, and learn how to cope with it.

Continuing Treatment Sessions

The main aspects of Erik's treatment included cognitive restructuring, in-session role plays of anxiety-provoking situations, and *in vivo* (real-life) exposures to anxiety-provoking situations, whereby Erik would actively practice doing the things that made him anxious. The cognitive and behavioral components of treatment were complementary in that they worked on both how to change his type of thinking by testing negative expectations and by accurately interpreting his successful social experiences (see Otto & Safren, 2000; Rapee & Heimberg, 1997). Cognitive restructuring for social anxiety is similar to cognitive restructuring for depression, as outlined in Chapter 4. Typically, to prevent the client from being overwhelmed, CBT for SAD begins with a situation that is lower on the fear hierarchy. An example of a situation higher on Erik's hierarchy is presented to illustrate better the crux of his presenting problem.

To "restructure" Erik's thinking, he and his therapist systematically reviewed the list of his thoughts and identified whether there were other, reasonable ways of interpreting the situation. They did this by looking at a list of typical cognitive distortions (e.g., "all-or-nothing thinking," "mind reading"), and using a list of questions to ask about each thought that would help to evaluate them (e.g., "What is the evidence that this is actually true?", "What is the evidence that it might not be true?", "Is there an alternate explanation?", "What would you say to a friend who is in a similar situation?"). An abridged version of a cognitive-restructuring dialogue the therapist had with Erik relative to the described situation follows:

THERAPIST: OK, so the gist of your thought process is that if you tried to talk to this guy, you would be anxious and therefore not be able to have a conversation; he would see that you are anxious, think you are a loser, and you would therefore never be able to meet anyone, ever.

ERIK: Yes.

THERAPIST: That is certainly putting a lot at stake in one conversation.

ERIK: Well, it's just that if I can't even have a conversation, how am I ever going to meet someone?

THERAPIST: I see what you are saying. And I can also see that if anyone had beliefs like this about conversations, they too would also avoid them and feel really terrible about a conversation, if they thought it didn't go well.

ERIK: Exactly.

THERAPIST: So, let's think about this a little more. The first thought is that if you are anxious, then you will not be able to have a conversation. Let's evaluate this thought first.

ERIK: Okay.

THERAPIST: How much do you believe this thought?

ERIK: I don't know. Ninety percent, I guess.

THERAPIST: OK. And what makes you think this thought is true?

ERIK: I just know it is. Every time I get anxious in conversations, I can't think of anything to say.

THERAPIST: OK. Well, let's look at what we have for evidence of this. Think back to your first appointment with me. Were you nervous coming into this appointment?

ERIK: Definitely.

THERAPIST: Right. I think you told me that before. So before coming into my office, if you were to rate your anxiety about coming in to therapy and talking about your problems with me, what would you rate it, on a scale from 0 to 100?

ERIK: It was pretty high. I mean, I did not know what to expect. I was not sure whether you would like me. And, I thought that these problems were so weird that you would think I was a loser.

THERAPIST: So your anxiety was pretty high.

ERIK: I guess so. Maybe about 90% or so.

THERAPIST: So, your anxiety was very high, in fact, almost as high as it could be.

ERIK: Right.

THERAPIST: And when the therapy session started, I asked you about your difficulties, and you were able to have the conversation and tell me about them.

ERIK: Yes, I guess that is true.

THERAPIST: And you were anxious the whole time?

ERIK: Well, I was more anxious at the beginning, but less so as it went on.

THERAPIST: OK, great. This is a major thing to remember. *Even though you were very anxious, you were still able to have the conversation*, answer all of my questions, and even ask some questions on your own.

ERIK: That's true, I guess.

THERAPIST: And you also noticed that your anxiety started out high but decreased as the conversation went on.

The therapist used this discussion to dispute the key automatic thoughts about Erik's association between being anxious and not being able to have conversations. At the end, they eventually developed the rational response, "I can still have a conversation even if I am anxious," which Erik was to test in further situations that caused anxiety. For this particular conversation, however, they also similarly restructured the other key automatic thought—that a conversation going poorly would indicate that Erik would never be able to have successful conversations. Erik's homework was actually to meet this man with the goal of introducing himself, saying his name, asking the guy three questions about himself, and answering any questions the guy asked him. After doing the exposure, Erik worked on ways to consider the experience a success. The therapist tried to point out that a success would be related to whether he met his goals, but not necessarily to the outcome of the situation (e.g., in this case, whether he went and introduced himself, but not whether they ended up going on a date), which was not completely in Erik's control.

Throughout the remainder of the treatment, Erik and his therapist used a similar strategy to help him continue to approach progressively more and more situations that caused him anxiety. His goal was to find other, gay male friends. Therefore, they continued to practice ways to prepare in advance for having conversations and, eventually, for Erik to attend gay-related social events.

In fact, behavioral exposures with cognitive restructuring preparation and postprocessing became overt goals of weekly practice: Erik put himself in situations in which he would have to practice having a conversation even if he was anxious. He and his therapist did simulated role-play conversations in the sessions themselves, where Erik could practice conversations and rate his anxiety as the role play continued. Once, the therapist had a colleague participate in the role play, because Erik quickly became habituated to practicing conversations with the therapist (i.e., the therapist no longer made him anxious). Slowly, he learned through actual experience—inside and outside of the sessions and cognitive restructuring—that he could have conversations even if he was anxious. Consequently, he gradually became less concerned with the added fear of having anxiety in a social situation (vs. fearing the social situation itself), then gradually experienced less fear in social situations.

Summary: Social Anxiety Disorder and the Case of Erik

The main parts of conducting CBT for SAD include psychoeducation, cognitive restructuring, and behavioral exposures. In conducting CBT for SAD with LGB individuals, the main tenets of CBT remain the same, but, because of potential differences in the development of same-sex sexual orientation in a predominately heterosexual society, therapists should be particularly aware of the potential for excessive anxiety in situations associated with same-sex attractions. In the case of Erik, these techniques began with almost the sole emphasis on dating and meeting friends. He gradually attended a gay-related social group and began to make friendships. At the end of the short-term treatment, Erik had the goal of using his new skills to begin working on his career on his own.

GENERALIZED ANXIETY DISORDER

Cognitive-Behavioral Assessment

After the general assessment and diagnosis of GAD, the therapist began to establish a functional analysis of Anna's worry, as well as indicators of its severity. To establish a baseline level of anxiety, Anna and her therapist used the Hamilton Anxiety Scale (Hamilton, 1959), a widely used clinician-administered rating scale. It contains a list of 14 symptoms of anxiety, with descriptors of each anxiety level. They used the scale at the beginning, midpoint, and toward the end of treatment.

Weekly, Anna completed the Beck Anxiety Inventory (BAI; Beck et al., 1988), and the Penn State Worry Questionnaire (Meyer, Miller, Metzger, & Borkovec, 1990) to monitor her progress. These scales confirmed high levels of anxiety and worry—to the point that she endorsed the highest ratings on almost all of the worry items on the Penn State scale (e.g., "Once I start worrying, I can't stop," "I worry all the time"). She also experienced significant physiological symptoms of anxiety (as reported on the BAI), such as "heart racing," "nervous," and "hands trembling." When questioned about "nervous" she reported that she was always restless and got tense muscles and headaches. From these assessments, the therapist made a list of the major topics of worry—and added items to the list that were not necessarily on the scale. Additionally, the use of the scales pointed to many of the somatic symptoms of anxiety, as well as poor "anxiety hygiene"—such as working on anxiety-provoking schoolwork until late hours of the evening and not being able to sleep, and excessive use of caffeine. Anna displayed a moderate-to-severe level of anxiety and worry according to each assessment.

Moving from Assessment to Treatment

Self-monitoring of symptoms is key to both treatment and assessment of GAD. Anna's therapist requested that she monitor her worry with a "worry notebook." Because Anna had already discussed problems with procrastination, a thorough discussion of the rationale for the CBT homework was essential (this discussion took up most of the second session). The therapist explained that this monitoring system would assist in helping her in several ways. Monitoring could (1) eventually reduce her anxiety, (2) identify a true sense of how frequently and intensely she was worrying, (3) help her learn about the triggers of her worry, (4) help her learn about the most frequent and interfering topics, and (5) help her learn when she would have relief.

    With Anna, the therapist also discussed the importance of making sure to actually do the notebook versus fretting about doing it perfectly, which could result in procrastinating and not doing it at all.

THERAPIST: So after talking about keeping a worry notebook, what do you think could get in the way of actually doing it?

ANNA: Well, knowing me, I would probably freak out about it, try to do it perfectly, and then put it off.

THERAPIST: OK, so it sounds like you have gotten pretty good at figuring out what the pattern seems to be.

ANNA: Hey, I am the one that lives with it.

THERAPIST: So we really need to problem-solve about how you might approach this task differently.

ANNA: I guess so.

THERAPIST: So, knowing in advance, do you have any ideas?

ANNA: Well, it's not like I am getting graded at school for this, so I suppose I could just really try to make sure just to put down what I am thinking, without overanalyzing it too much.

THERAPIST: I think that's a great point. As we continue to work together, I think we need to keep in mind the different approaches you take. We can call what you might have done in the past, the "old way." Because we know that the "old way" doesn't really work the way you want, let's call this new strategy the "new way," and see how it works out.

In this respect, the CBT homework can act as practice for many of the other areas in which a patient may have difficulty. With respect to the self-monitoring, Anna and the therapist decided it would make the most sense to break down the days into four time periods: (1) morning (before leaving the house), (2) morning at school, (3) afternoon, and (4) evening. For each time period, Anna would denote the antecedent—the trigger or situation (see Chapter 2); the behavior—the topic of her worry/worry thoughts, and her level of worry/anxiety (subjective 1–10-point scale); and the consequence—what ended up happening as a result/what she did afterwards. During the time periods, she could also record how long the worry episode lasted and, if the need arose, put more than one episode in each time period.

As is evident from the worry notebook (Figure 5.4) and other issues described, Anna's presenting problem, generalized anxiety, was not directly related to her sexual orientation. However, her relationship with her girlfriend was compromised, and her parents' pressure on her to find a husband contributed to her anxiety. After monitoring and completion of 1 week of the worry notebook, the therapist and Anna further discussed the three components of anxiety and how it related to her presenting problems (Figure 5.5). This was also used to help her stay motivated with the treatment and to understand the rationale.

Continuing Treatment Sessions

Anna's treatment was based on traditional cognitive-behavioral approaches to GAD (e.g., Newman & Borkovec, 1995; Zinbarg et al., 1993). The information from the assessment guided the case conceptu-

Tuesday morning

　Antecedent: *I don't know, I just woke up anxious.*

　Topics: *I am never going to get everything done that I need to today, I am overwhelmed. My life sucks. I am never going to graduate from social work school. I am going to end up working in a bookstore again.*

　Level of worry (1–10): *9*

　How long it lasted: *Until I got to school.*

　Consequence (what did you do afterwards?): *Gave one-word answers to Sarah when she asked me questions, had an argument about her thinking that I am being mean to her.*

Tuesday morning at school

　Antecedent: *I was not really worrying during this morning at school. Went to class, sat with classmates—just occasional worries here and there.*

　Topics: *Not sure whether I got everything down that the teacher was saying in class.*

　Level of worry (1–10): *2*

　How long it lasted: *Until I got to school.*

　Consequence (what did you do afterwards?): *Nothing*

Tuesday afternoon

　Antecedent: *Free time between two classes*

　Topics: *What should I be doing now to be productive? I need to use my time wisely. I have 2 hours, and I could be accomplishing a lot right now. Where do I begin?*

　Level of worry (1–10): 7

　How long it lasted: *Until my next class started.*

　Consequence (what did you do afterwards?): *I did not get much done, because I spent the whole time worrying too much. Ended up smoking cigarettes and drinking coffee.*

Tuesday evening

　Antecedent: *Arrived home*

　Topics: *What should I do first? I have to make dinner. Sarah is going to be home soon, and I need to spend time with her, but I am so behind with schoolwork. I can't believe I got myself into this situation. Not only am I going to end up with a shitty job, but I will also end up alone, because I am going to mess up my relationship.*

　Level of worry (1–10): *8*

　How long it lasted: *All night—off an on.*

　Consequence (what did you do afterwards?): *Didn't end up making dinner as I had thought I would, called friends to commiserate about schoolwork, tried to write one paper for an incomplete but did not know where to begin, stayed up till about midnight, alternated between reading and sitting at the computer. Couldn't fall asleep.*

FIGURE 5.4. Sample worry notebook entry for Anna (generalized anxiety disorder).

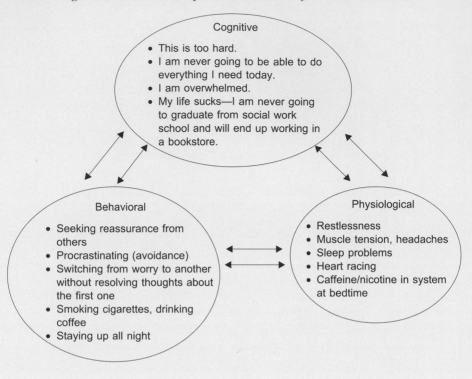

Cognitive

- This is too hard.
- I am never going to be able to do everything I need today.
- I am overwhelmed.
- My life sucks—I am never going to graduate from social work school and will end up working in a bookstore.

Behavioral

- Seeking reassurance from others
- Procrastinating (avoidance)
- Switching from worry to another without resolving thoughts about the first one
- Smoking cigarettes, drinking coffee
- Staying up all night

Physiological

- Restlessness
- Muscle tension, headaches
- Sleep problems
- Heart racing
- Caffeine/nicotine in system at bedtime

FIGURE 5.5. Anna's thoughts, behaviors, and physical symptoms.

alization and treatment, which included a variety of skills aimed at reduction of anxiety and coping with worry. These included training in cognitive restructuring, worry delay, and worry exposure with response prevention (the response was reassurance seeking), and, on her own, relaxation training.

Seeking reassurance is a typical behavioral component of GAD, and the target was mainly Anna's partner. This part of her treatment can be referred to as "exposure with response prevention," or ERP. This method for treating anxiety disorders is to help the patient habituate to her fears by exposing her to them, but preventing the typical response (i.e., Foa & Kozac, 1986). The response—in this case, reassurance seeking—typically reinforces the actual behavior of worry in that it does not allow for habituation. The approach is similar to treatment of any other anxiety disorder or phobia; however, for GAD, worries only occur in one's head, and it therefore makes it harder to face the feared situation head on. For example, in treating someone with OCD who compulsively washes his hands, the patient would be exposed to an anxiety provoking stimulus, say something dirty. The "response prevention" would be that the patient would not be allowed to wash his hands and would eventually habituate to the anxiety that ensued. For a height phobic, the treatment is to take the client to different heights and to prevent the response (leaving) until his or her anxiety decreases. For GAD, it is important to figure out whether there are typical responses— though they may be more subtle—and help the patient learn to prevent these responses and habituate to his or her anxiety.

Because Sarah, Anna's partner, was one of the main foci of her reassurance seeking, the therapist suggested that Sarah join them for one session. Sarah had much to say about Anna's reassurance seeking.

SARAH: The main thing I wanted to tell you about is the amount of time Anna spends "processing" her worries with other people.

ANNA: I do not.

THERAPIST: Let's let Sarah explain. Remember, the main point here is to be honest, and to try to figure out how to best help you.

SARAH: Sorry, Anna, but it's true. It seems like from the time you get home from work, you first talk to me about the different worries you are having, then call your mother and talk to her about it for a couple of hours, then usually talk to at least one other friend about it until late at night. It's really bad (*turning to therapist*). I mean, usually she is worrying about and complaining about schoolwork, and getting people to tell her it will be OK, but if she spent one-fourth of the time she talks about it actually *doing* it, she would be done. Then, when we are together and she is not on the phone, she is just always irritable.

THERAPIST: Anna, do you think this is true—that you spend a lot of time discussing your worries with other people?

ANNA: I think Sarah is exaggerating, but I think I do talk a lot on the phone about it. And when I am not talking about, I am just worrying in my head most of the time.

THERAPIST: This is a really important thing, and I am glad it got brought up. I want to refer back to something that Anna and I have discussed in the past. This is the fact that anxiety usually maintains itself because of a cycle of different types of thoughts and behaviors. This behavior we are talking about here—you have called it "processing" your worries with other people—is talking about it. I am going to use a different word for it. I am going to call it "getting reassurance."

ANNA: I definitely need to do that a lot.

THERAPIST: Well, here is the thing. From what I gather, even though it feels good in the moment, it may actually not help you that much—in fact, I think that reassurance actually makes the anxiety worse.

ANNA: How so?

THERAPIST: Well, here is the thing (*points back to three-circle model of anxiety*). Remember when we constructed this model?

ANNA: Yes.

THERAPIST: Well, let me also show it to Sarah. I am just going to focus on two of the circles here. In the circle labeled "cognitive" we have worries such as "This is too hard," "I am never going to be able to do it," and so on. Because of these worries, Sarah, and many other people who have anxiety problems, go to other people for reassurance. This is a behavior—and it is in the circle labeled behavioral "reassurance seeking." Because people generally make her feel better by telling her, "Oh, you can do it" or "It won't be as bad as you think" Anna then feels better in the moment.

ANNA: So, if it feels better, why would it be bad?

THERAPIST: Well, there are several reasons. First, by spending so much time speaking with other people, you never get the chance to actually do the schoolwork you are worrying about, you never get the chance to *learn* you can do it, and you never get the chance to learn that you do not *need* to seek reassurance from others. Second, by asking for reassurance and getting it, you are becoming more and more dependent on other people to make you feel OK about your abilities, and it gets harder and harder to do things on your own.

SARAH: I had a feeling you were going to say something like this.

ANNA: But this is the main thing that gets me through the day.

THERAPIST: I am not saying this is going to be easy—I am just saying that this is something we need to work on. I think you will find that, over time, as you cut back on seeking reassurance, you will slowly have the need less and less, and in fact, in conjunction with the other things we work on, you will slowly worry less and less. The hard thing is the beginning, when you have to really work hard at not getting reassurance and sit with the anxiety you feel—instead of going for the instantly gratifying solution of getting reassurance and feeling better.

SARAH: So how do I fit in?

THERAPIST: Well, from my perspective, I think that Anna is going to have to agree to try to ask for reassurance less and less from you and other people. Sarah, when Anna does ask you for reassurance, I think you will need to just say, "We agreed not to talk about things like this." And Anna, you are going to have to agree to not get mad at Sarah when she responds this way.

Although Anna was reluctant to reduce her reassurance seeking, she agreed to give it a try. The information presented here was not a complete surprise to Anna, because she and her therapist had previously discussed it during the explanation of the model of anxiety at the beginning of treatment. Sarah, Anna's partner, really found this useful and felt that it would significantly improve their relationship.

To help Anna cut back on reassurance seeking and other behavioral components of anxiety, she learned cognitive restructuring procedures. The training in cognitive restructuring for GAD follows an approach similar to that described in the cases of social anxiety and depression, and is therefore not described in detail here. In this instance, Anna learned how to identify and list thoughts from her worry notebook, and to go through a process of disputing them and coming up with a rational response. Because the worry notebook revealed that mornings were particularly fraught with worry for her, the therapist and Anna collaboratively decided that Anna would start her day with cognitive restructuring, right before breakfast. Although the cognitive restructuring did not directly target Anna's behavior toward her partner, Sarah, they eventually found that, after doing the exercise regularly, Anna's perceived need to seek reassurance from her partner began to decrease, and they were able to have more positive interactions.

After using cognitive restructuring and cutting back on reassurance seeking for a several weeks, Anna learned "worry delay" and "worry exposure" techniques. The therapist and Anna worked together to develop a system for dealing with worry when cognitive restructuring did not work. Anna would write down her worry in the notebook and distinctly tell herself that she would worry about it later. Every night, she would then pick several of these worries and specifically focus on them; although at first her anxiety went up, it eventually came back down. In focusing on the worries, generally, patients are instructed to come up with vivid images, and not to become distracted. This was difficult for Anna; therefore, she and her therapist worked on one example in session, in which they wrote out one of her worst fears, then read the description into a tape recorder. Anna then would listen to the tape and concentrate on it until her anxiety would go down. This method also allowed for exposure with response prevention, in that Anna would be able to habituate to the anxiety, without responding by getting reassurance or distracting herself with either a new worry or another set of thoughts. This typically took her about 20 minutes. Recall that Anna had worries about schoolwork, but she also felt that some of these worries were related to her feelings of inadequacy as a person, because of her sexual orientation. An example of the worry situation that they recorded on tape in session, which includes both of these issues, follows:

> "Picture yourself at home, trying to concentrate on your schoolwork. Picture what your apartment and room look like; picture yourself at your desk, attempting to study. Focus on what it all looks like, what it smells like. . . . You are thinking to yourself, 'I can't do this,' 'I am overwhelmed.' As you try to do your work, you realize that you really cannot do it, that the material is too difficult, that there is too much of it, and that you cannot possibly imagine completing it all.
>
> "It's now 6 months later, the time when you would have graduated from social work school. You are sitting in the graduation, but not with the other students. Picture each student slowly going up and getting his or her diploma. You are not one of them. Your are by yourself in the audience watching, because you did not complete all of the work. Notice what it feels like as each person gets his or her diploma, what the room looks like, what others are saying and doing. All the time, however, you know that you did not complete the work, and you are not going to graduate.
>
> "Picture yourself telling your father that you were not able to complete the work. Picture what it would be like to speak with him, the look on his face as you explain the problem, and how it has nothing to do with his disappointment about you also being a lesbian. Imagine yourself having to have this conversation with him and what it would be like."

The text of the worry exposure illustrates one of the central themes of this book—that sexual orientation is a component of CBT with LGB clients, but not necessarily the primary component of it. Anna was a patient suffering from GAD, and her treatment followed general principles of CBT. However, sexual orientation did play a role, in that her fear of lack of success was linked to a general fear of not living up to her father's standards—related to both educational achievement and Anna's choice of a female partner.

Cognitive restructuring, worry exposure/worry delays, and monitoring with the worry notebook were the main skills employed for cognitive-behavioral management of Anna's anxiety symptoms. For GAD treatment, relaxation training is also typically employed to help with excessive autonomic arousal. The relaxation training typically involves a 20-minute procedure, whereby clients progressively tense and relax each major muscle group. In this case, to maximize the use of sessions, Anna purchased a relaxation tape, which she used on her own. This helped her with both sleep and in dealing with anxiety symptoms throughout the day.

Gradually, Anna decreased her worry behaviors and used much of the time that she had spent on them more functionally—actually doing the schoolwork. She became better at concentrating during times when she wanted to do her schoolwork. This allowed her to enjoy her leisure time instead of spending it worrying about work. Anna continued to have a tendency to worry more than most people; however, after treatment, she felt that she could control this better. Although the core of her treatment took place over 20 weekly sessions, Anna required subsequent monthly booster sessions over the course of a year.

Chapter 6

Couple Therapies

This chapter presents three models of cognitive and behavioral couple therapy, and discusses their adaptation to the treatment of same-sex couples. The vast majority of the literature on couple therapy presumes that the couple being treated is heterosexual (and most presume that couples are also married), so much of this chapter focuses on a review of cognitive and behavioral approaches to treating relationship distress developed with heterosexual couples as the target treatment population. Regardless of sexual orientation, many of the issues faced by distressed couples are quite similar, and treatment approaches developed for heterosexual couples can often be used effectively to treat same-sex couples, with little or no modification. However, some issues unique to same-sex couples must be taken into consideration and are also addressed here.

Before beginning our discussion of therapy with same-sex couples, some cautions are in order regarding limitations of the available empirical data. First, because none of the major outcome studies reviewed here included sexual orientation as a demographic variable, the approaches described in this chapter have yet to be empirically validated for same-sex couples. Second, whereas there is a paucity of literature on same-sex couple therapy, even less is known about the special concerns facing ethnic minority individuals in same-sex relationships. The multiple minority group membership and identity issues experienced by ethnic minority gay men and lesbians may create unique relationship strains in addition to those experienced by nonminority couples. Given the complexity of these issues and the paucity of available research data, the issue of ethnic minority status among gay and lesbian couples is not addressed here.[1] The reader should be aware that much of the research on same-sex couples has been conducted with white, middle-class participants, with limited extrapolation to other demographic groups.

GARY AND WALTER: NEGOTIATING POWER AND INTIMACY

Gary and Walter, a gay, male couple, had been together for 10 years and were 16 years apart in age. Walter had a career in sales and a significantly larger income than Gary, who worked as an aide in a retirement home. Both described Walter, age 50, as the "dominant" partner, and Walter went on to say that he felt like a "father figure" to Gary. Both felt that, in recent years, they had begun to grow apart, and particularly in the past 6 months, they had become increasingly distant, with Gary moving to the downstairs bedroom about a month prior to therapy. They were coming to therapy to "try to get some help before giving up." Their search for a therapist was precipitated by a crisis about a month earlier, when Gary found out that Walter had answered a personal ad, had gone on three dates with another man, and had been sexual with this person. Gary and Walter had discussed the possibility of non-monogamy in their relationship, but this had been some years earlier, and the topic had not been revisited since. Gary felt that Walter had deceived him by having a sexual relationship with another man.

Both partners identified poor communication as a major problem in their relationship. Gary admitted to not "fighting fair" and acknowledged that he often said provocative things during arguments, such as threatening to leave the relationship. He also tended to be very critical of Walter and had trouble staying on one topic, often bringing up old hurts and conflicts. Although Gary recognized that some of his behavior during arguments was not constructive, he also said that when he was angry "at least he had Walter's attention." On his part, Walter was a self-described "poor communicator." During arguments, he tended to withdraw, both in the moment by becoming "stony and silent," and also by retreating to another room or leaving the house. Due to their style of communicating, problems rarely got resolved, and both felt that they had many resentments stored up over the years.

JULIA AND ELLIE: "WHAT DO LESBIANS BRING TO THEIR SECOND DATE?"

Julia and Ellie, a lesbian couple, had been together for 4 years. Overall, they reported a high level of satisfaction with their relationship, but they related that in the year prior to entering therapy, they had hit a "rough spot" that eventually led to Julia's moving out, and they were separated for about 2 months. They had recently gotten back together and were seeking therapy to strengthen their relationship and to avoid "making the same mistakes" that led to their separation.

Julia and Ellie met while both were working for the same company, and struck up a friendship that quickly become romantic when both expressed attraction for one another after a couple of months. Ellie had been married to a man and was recently divorced when she met Julia, who had identified as lesbian since she was a teenager. Although Julia had dated women for many years, she had not had long-term relationships with a woman until becoming involved with Ellie; this was the first lesbian relationship for Ellie. As with some lesbian couples, Julia and Ellie's relationship reached a high level of commitment soon after they got together. The early phase of their relationship was characterized by a high degree of closeness, sexual compatibility, and intensity. They moved in together after 6 months, and both described this early phase of their relationship as intensely intimate and rewarding. However, in retrospect, both felt that they had committed to one another and moved in together very quickly. Ellie, in particular, felt that she had not taken enough time to process her divorce and her newly recognized attraction to women. Some friends teased Julia and Ellie that they were fulfilling the lesbian stereotype depicted in the joke, "What do lesbians bring to their second date? A U-Haul."

About a year into their relationship, the couple's insularity and dependence on one another were further heightened when Ellie lost her job and they decided to move to Seattle together to look for new work. In the new city, Julia quickly found a job, but Ellie remained unemployed for some time and became increasingly depressed. Furthermore, neither woman had many friends in Seattle, and both missed the support network they'd formed in the other city. Eventually, Ellie found work, and both began making some friends, but in the year prior to entering therapy, both said that their relationship began to deteriorate. Julia particularly felt increasingly irritated with Ellie and "picked fights" with her about seemingly inconsequential topics, after which the couple would withdraw and not speak to one another for several hours. As Julia felt increasingly less connected with Ellie, she began to seek connection elsewhere and started spending more and more time with friends. Their sex life diminished, and both said that they began to feel like "roommates" rather than partners.

In addition to the stressors they were experiencing within their relationship, Julia and Ellie had very little social support as a lesbian couple. Although they were out to some of their nonwork friends, they did not come out to colleagues at work, which contributed to their feeling of isolation. Neither had made any gay or lesbian friends in the new city. Also, while Ellie's family was somewhat accepting of their relationship, Julia's family was not. Her mother made frequent comments about "never having grandchildren" (Julia's sister, her only sibling, was already married and had decided not to have children). When Julia reminded her mother that it was quite possible for a lesbian couple to have children, her mother retorted, "In that case, I'd rather not have any grandkids." Julia's family was also not accepting of Ellie as Julia's primary significant other. The couple discovered this after Julia had minor surgery during their first year together, and her family told Ellie that they would be making all of the decisions regarding Julia's care in case of emergency.

Three months prior to therapy, Julia decided to move out, and she got her own apartment. Julia said that Ellie was supportive of her move, which she took as an indication that Ellie didn't want to be with her any more. Although Julia felt that moving out was "the right thing to do," she says that she quickly became "miserable" in her new apartment and missed Ellie intensely. They talked by phone and e-mail, eventually deciding to get back together on the condition that they seek couple therapy to help them deal with the issues that had led to their separation.

ISSUES UNIQUE TO SAME-SEX COUPLES

The couples presented in the case examples are dealing with many issues that are not unique to same-sex couples. Research indicates that the correlates of relationship satisfaction are similar between same-sex and heterosexual couples (e.g., Kurdek, 1995), and that levels of relationship satisfaction are also comparable (Green, Bettinger, & Zachs, 1996). Communication difficulties, conflict resolution, and balancing closeness and independence are common problems for couples regardless of sexual orientation, and the cognitive and behavioral approaches described here are just as applicable for same-sex couples facing these problems as for heterosexual couples. However, several unique issues are more likely to have an impact on gay and lesbian couples, and it is critical for therapists working with this population to take these issues into consideration in assessment, case conceptualization, and as potential foci for therapeutic interventions.

Negative Bias and Discrimination

Perhaps the most salient problem facing same-sex couples and distinguishing them from their heterosexual counterparts is the experience of homo-negative bias and discrimination (e.g., Green & Mitchell, 2002). Most LGB individuals have faced or will face negative bias at some time in their lives. Negative bias and homophobia can occur at a variety of levels, including within one's family of origin, in the workplace, and at a larger cultural and societal level. Discriminatory behavior as a result of negative bias and homophobia may take many forms, including overt harassment and violence, being fired from jobs or overlooked for promotion, as well as more subtle forms, such as the lack of positive representation of gay individuals and couples in the media (Ossana, 2000). Furthermore, although internalized homophobia is a controversial concept and may not be as pervasive as was once believed (e.g., Meyer & Dean, 1998), there is certainly evidence to suggest that living in a nonsupportive-to-hostile social milieu can undermine lesbian and gay individuals' self-esteem and well-being (e.g., Hancock, 2000).

In addition to their impact on individual functioning, homophobia and discrimination can have various effects on same-sex couples. Exposure to negative stereotypes depicting gay and lesbian individuals as hypersexual, and their relationships as short-lived, can lead to doubts regarding the viability of long-term same-sex relationships (Ossana, 2000). Such doubts are increased by the fact that LGB couples may no longer frequent bars and other social gatherings, choosing rather to create stable homes, and are therefore less visible as representatives of successful couples. The institution of marriage provides a social and legal sanctioning of heterosexual, committed relationships that is not available to gay and lesbian couples. Although same-sex couples may choose to create a ritual of their own by having a formal commitment ceremony, they are still not afforded the numerous, substantial legal and financial benefits available to married (or, in many cases, cohabiting unmarried) heterosexual couples in the U.S. and most parts of the world (Kuehlwein & Gottschalk, 2000). Legislated discrimination also restricts access to other privileges that are automatically granted to heterosexual individuals, including an absence of legal protection for same-sex partners in child-custody battles and restrictions on the ability to make important medical decisions about one's partner.

Homo-negative bias and discrimination can also have an effect on the couple's social integration and support. Such negative responses in one or both partners' families of origin may make integrating one's partner into one's biological family more challenging. Fear of homophobic responses makes coming out to family, friends, and coworkers a stressful decision for many gay and lesbian individuals, and differences between partners regarding how much and to whom to be out can be a source of conflict. The degree to which the couple is "out" in turn has an impact on their available social support and degree of isolation. For example, a couple who is not out to friends and coworkers may experience considerable stress related to keeping the relationship a secret, may have few or no models for healthy same-sex relationships, and may be deprived of the usual benefits of being able to talk about problems experienced in a primary relationship.

Cognitive and behavioral therapies for same-sex couples are well suited to address these issues. For example, therapy can help members of couples communicate clearly to one another about coming-out issues, including discussion of the meaning, impact, and pros and cons of coming out for each partner. Emotional acceptance interventions can be particularly useful when there are differences between partners in the degree to which each wants to or has come out in various settings. Cognitive interventions can help partners examine their internalized beliefs about the viability of same-sex committed relationships, and how those beliefs may in turn influence the choices they make regarding their own union. Therapy can provide a forum for couples to choose and create their own rituals. In addition, therapy can provide external validation of their relationship that is often unavailable to same-sex couples in the broader social context. Finally, therapists can point the way to gay and lesbian affirmative reading materials and community resources.

Bisexuality

Bisexual individuals in same-sex relationships may not only face many of the issues discussed in this section but may also face additional issues that may impede their relationship functioning. One or both partners identifying as bisexual has implications for issues of commitment and monogamy. Some studies have indicated that bisexuals are more likely than gay men or lesbians to prefer a sexually non-monogamous relationship (Rust, 1996). The same-sex partner of a bisexual individual may experience insecurity regarding the possibility of losing his or her partner not only to someone of the same gender but also to someone of the opposite gender. A gay or lesbian individual may view his or her partner's bisexuality as an indication of diminished commitment to the relationship or to a gay identity. Furthermore, in addition to the homophobia experienced by many sexual minority individuals, bisexual individuals may experience an additional lack of acceptance from the gay and lesbian community.

The therapist working with couples in which one or both partners identify as bisexual can help the couple to communicate clearly and honestly regarding their level of relationship commitment and desire for sexual exclusivity. Furthermore, CBT can be helpful to explore underlying "biphobic" assumptions or beliefs held by a bisexual individual about him- or herself, or by a gay man or lesbian about his or her bisexual partner. Finally, the therapist can provide validation for their relationship and recommend resources in the community, such as bisexual support groups.

Gender-Role Socialization

Much has been written about the impact of gender-role socialization on the functioning of same-sex couples. Some theorists have argued that relationships consisting of two men or two women represent a sort of "socialization squared" (Ossana, 2000), in which the primary strengths and attributes of the couple's gender are overrepresented, whereas strengths of the other gender are underrepresented. Specifically, because men are socialized to value independence, achievement, and instrumentality, it is thought that gay male couples excel in these areas but have difficulty forming close, intimate bonds. In contrast, women are socialized to value relationships and intimacy; therefore, it is thought that women in lesbian relationships become overly bonded or "merged," while having difficulty maintaining autonomy.

Although this view has been widely held among clinicians working with same-sex couples, it is predicated on several assumptions that have not received consistent empirical support. First, it assumes that gender-role socialization is the same for gay and lesbian youths as for heterosexual youths. There is some evidence, however, that this is not the case. For example, lesbians and gay men reported that they were significantly less conforming to traditional gender roles in childhood than were heterosexual men and women (Green et al., 1996). Furthermore, Kurdek (1987) found that the self-concepts of adult lesbians and gay men incorporated more of the opposite gender's attributes than did the self-concepts of their heterosexual counterparts: Lesbians' self-concepts included more instrumentality than those of heterosexual women, whereas gay men's self-concepts included more expressiveness than those of heterosexual men. First, because these findings indicate that gender-role socialization may not operate in the same way for gay men and lesbians, they call into question the "socialization squared" view of same-sex relationships. Second, this view is also predicated on the belief that an abundance of one or the other set of attributes is inherently problematic. Again, this assumption is not necessarily accurate and has not consistently been borne out by empirical data. For example, some data indicate that the high degree of intimacy achieved by some lesbian couples is associated with high self-reported levels of relationship satisfaction (Green et al., 1996).

Rather than assuming that gay male relationships automatically lack intimacy or that lesbian relationships inevitably have difficulty with autonomy, the therapist's goal in therapy with same-sex couples is to help them find a healthy balance between intimacy and autonomy, a struggle that is also common among heterosexual couples. Furthermore, perhaps a strength of same-sex couples is that, because they cannot fall back on traditional division of roles along gender lines, they have to create their own balance. Research shows that most same-sex couples desire egalitarian relationships, and that sharing both instrumental and expressive roles is associated with relationship satisfaction (Carrington, 1999; Kurdek & Schmitt, 1986). As in the earlier case examples, the cognitive-behavioral couple therapist can help couples examine their own assumptions about gender roles in general and in their particular partnership, resolve conflicts around division of labor, and address differences in desired levels of intimacy and autonomy.

Differing Relationship Norms

It is important for therapists working with same-sex couples to be aware of heterosexist biases and not to assume that normative behavior in heterosexual relationships is necessarily normative to the same extent in same-sex relationships. Perhaps the most prominent observed difference in norms is the issue of monogamy. Among the majority of heterosexual and lesbian couples, sex outside of the primary relationship is often viewed as a form of betrayal, disloyalty, and lack of commitment to the relationship. In fact, in traditional behavioral couple therapy, a clinician working with a heterosexual couple in which an affair is taking place might even refuse to commence treatment until the affair is discontinued. In contrast, sexual non-monogamy among gay men is a frequent and accepted occurrence (e.g., Blumstein & Schwartz, 1983; McWhirter & Mattison, 1984). Gay men are apt to view sex outside of the relationship as purely recreational, and often define their relationship in terms of emotional commitment and fidelity rather than sexual exclusivity. Furthermore, for many gay men choosing to open up the relationship can be a political statement, one way of rejecting traditional cultural norms that have been oppressive to them (Greenan & Tunnell, 2003). A number of studies have found comparable levels of relationship satisfaction among sexually monogamous versus non-monogamous gay couples (e.g., Blasband & Peplau, 1985; Blumstein & Schwartz, 1983). As in the case of Gary and Walter, it is often not sex outside of the relationship per se that is the problem, but issues of trust, power imbalance, lack of clarity about the parameters, and other challenges that cause conflict among non-monogamous gay male couples. The therapist working with gay male couples needs to evaluate the impact of outside sexual relationships within the norms of this community rather than applying heterosexual standards. That members of non-monogamous couples openly discuss such an arrangement is particularly important given the risk of contracting sexually transmitted diseases and infecting unwitting partners. If non-monogamy is treated as an adulterous secret to be maintained, the couple may actually increase health risks that could be avoided by honest discussion of a potentially difficult topic.

Although the issue of monogamy has received considerable focus, there are other areas in which the norms for gay and lesbian couples differ from those of their heterosexual counterparts. For example, lesbians are more likely to maintain close friendships with former partners than are heterosexual women, and "exes" often become a part of the couple's extended family (e.g., Clunis & Green, 2000). Friendship with former lovers can, however, cause problems in the current relationship, including the new partner feeling jealous or threatened by the emotional closeness and history shared between her partner and her partner's ex. As with the issue of non-monogamy, the therapist working with lesbian couples can help them to communicate clearly regarding their feelings about ex-partners and discuss the impact of friendships with exes on the current relationship. These issues underscore the importance of being aware of heterosexist biases when working with gay and lesbian couples. Rather than assuming that heterosexual relationship norms apply, the therapist working with same-sex couples should instead help them to clarify and communicate to one another about their own relationship rules and expectations.

Creating Families and Having Children

The issue of creating and maintaining a family for gay men and lesbians is complex and is dealt with in depth elsewhere (e.g., Matthews & Lease, 2000). For the purposes of this chapter, the main issue for therapists to keep in mind is that gay and lesbian couples often create, both by choice and by necessity, family constellations that differ from the traditional definition of family. Given negative responses to coming out in one's family of origin, gay men and lesbians often create a "chosen family," a group of non-biologically related individuals who form a close social network, and with whom the individual is often closer than he or she is to biological relatives. Where access to the social and legal institution of marriage is lacking, many gay and lesbian couples choose to formalize and honor their union with a commitment ceremony. It is important for the therapist working with same-sex couples to be aware of, encourage, and legitimize the ways in which gay and lesbian couples can create family and community.

Furthermore, more and more gay men and lesbians are choosing to become parents, and they do so in a great variety of ways.[2] Regardless of the path to parenthood, considerable research indicates that gay men and lesbians are just as adept at parenting as their heterosexual counterparts, and that children of gay and lesbian parents do not experience any greater psychological distress than do children of heterosexual parents (see Matthews & Lease, 2000, for an extensive review of issues involving LBG parenting).

Despite considerable evidence supporting their competency, gay and lesbian parents continue to face societal prejudice (e.g., McLeod & Crawford, 1998). This prejudice is expressed in a variety of ways. For example, gay and lesbian families are rarely portrayed in the media. Gay and lesbian parents of children from previous marriages may fear that custody or visitation rights will be taken away if their sexual orientation is discovered, and this fear is often justified, given negative legal precedents and a lack of legal protection for individuals in this situation. It is important for the therapist working with gay and lesbian parents to be aware of and validate these concerns. It is helpful for the therapist to be aware of the legal status of gay and lesbian families in his or her area, because laws regarding gay and lesbian families' rights differ considerably from state to state. Furthermore, the therapist can help clients find and make use of supportive community resources, such as therapy or social groups for gay and lesbian parents.

TRADITIONAL BEHAVIORAL COUPLE THERAPY: CHANGING PROBLEMATIC RELATIONSHIP BEHAVIORS

Regardless of sexual orientation, many couples come to therapy with some very similar relationship problems, including a paucity of positive interactions, difficulty with communication, and difficulty in effectively resolving conflicts. Traditional behavioral couple therapy (TBCT, also known as behavioral marital therapy; Jacobson & Margolin, 1979) was designed to address these deficits. TBCT adheres to a behavioral conceptualization of relationship distress, in which behavior is viewed as being maintained by environmental factors through the processes of operant and respondent conditioning. From a behavioral perspective, a couple's relationship is viewed as a series of continuous, reciprocal interactions, in which each partner's behavior is shaped and maintained by the other partner's responses. TBCT is firmly rooted in social learning theory, which posits a continual, reciprocal relationship between behavior and environment, and also suggests that the effect of environmental contingencies may be mediated by internal processes, including cognitions and emotions. TBCT is also linked to behavior exchange theory, which views all relationships as a constant exchange of positive and negative behaviors; in this view, relationship satisfaction is seen as directly related to the ratio of benefits and costs received in the relationship. TBCT is a change-based approach: Interventions focus on each partner changing his or her own behavior in ways that improve his or her partner's relationship satisfaction. Each partner is encouraged to acknowledge his or her role in problems and to unilaterally make changes that can increase relationship satisfaction, independent of any expectations of partner change. Because of this emphasis on each partner being willing and able to change his or her own behavior, TBCT requires a high degree of collaboration between partners. Therapists can explain this process to clients by emphasizing the difficulty in changing another's behavior, and the fact that if each partner agrees to change her or his behavior, the resultant improvement in the relationship may allow each partner to get what he or she desires.

Interventions in TBCT fall into three main categories: behavior exchange, communication training, and problem-solving training. *Behavior exchange* is based on the principle that in distressed couples, there is often an erosion of behaviors that were previously reinforcing, resulting in a low ratio of positive-to-negative behaviors and decreased relationship satisfaction. Behavior exchange helps couples to increase their exchange of positive, reinforcing behaviors deliberately. This is accomplished by having partners identify specific behaviors that are reinforcing to both the giver and the reciever of the behavior, and that are of relatively low emotional cost to the giver. Each partner then commits to engaging in one or more of these behaviors as a "homework assignment" between sessions; partners are also encouraged to reinforce one another for doing so. In *communication training*, couples' expressive and receptive communication skills are targeted. Partners are taught to express their own feelings and avoid blaming, and to improve their listening skills by paraphrasing their partners' statements, asking clarifying questions, and providing feedback. Partners practice these skills both in session and in between-session homework assignments. Finally, couples' ability to address successfully and resolve conflicts is improved through *problem-solving training*. Partners are taught a structured problem-solving format in which they learn to talk about only one problem at a time, clearly define the problem in nonblaming ways, take responsibility for their contribution to the problem, brainstorm potential solutions, implement an agreed-upon solution, and evaluate and modify the solution as needed. TBCT relies heavily on between-session homework assignments to generalize skills to the home environment. Through gradual fading of therapist prompts and the use of homework assignments, new behaviors acquired in therapy are gradually brought under the control of contingencies operating within the couple's relationship, rather than those contacted in the therapy setting.

TBCT is the most widely studied approach to treating relationship distress, and its efficacy has been demonstrated in over 20 randomized clinical trials (Baucom, Shoham, Meuser, Daiuto, & Stickle, 1998; Christensen & Heavey, 1999). However, these studies have also revealed significant limitations in both the clinical significance and the durability of improvements produced by TBCT. First, at least one-third of couples in randomized clinical trials of TBCT are treatment nonresponders and have not moved into the nondistressed range on standardized measures of marital satisfaction by the conclusion of treatment (Jacobson & Addis, 1993). Second, among those couples who do achieve clinically significant improvement, many do not maintain their gains and relapse to relationship distress at 2-year follow-up (Jacobson, Schmaling, & Holtzworth-Munroe, 1987).

One aspect of TBCT that may account for some of these limitations is that its effectiveness is predicated on a high degree of collaboration between partners. Because TBCT pushes for change from both partners, dyads that are less able or willing to compromise, collaborate, and accommodate one another are less likely to benefit from TBCT strategies. Jacobson and colleagues hypothesized that couples who are older, more disengaged, more traditional, and more polarized regarding important aspects of marital functioning are less likely to benefit from behavioral marital therapy than couples who are younger, more egalitarian, emotionally engaged, and whose views on what constitutes a healthy relationship are more similar (Jacobson & Christensen, 1996; Jacobson et al., 1987). Integrative behavioral couple therapy (IBCT; Jacobson & Christensen, 1996; Christensen & Jacobson, 2000) was developed to address some of the limitations of TBCT.

INTEGRATIVE BEHAVIORAL COUPLE THERAPY: ADDING ACCEPTANCE TO CHANGE STRATEGIES

IBCT adds to the traditional change strategies of TBCT an emphasis on emotional acceptance to help couples increase emotional intimacy even in the face of seemingly unsolvable problems. Although still rooted in behavioral principles, the goal of IBCT is to develop behaviors maintained by naturally occurring contingencies in the couple's relationship, rather than behaviors that are governed by the rules and instructions of therapy. IBCT is also designed to help couples become closer, even when change is not possible.

IBCT utilizes the change strategies of TBCT to some extent, but its emphasis is on emotional acceptance. Jacobson and Christensen (1996) define "acceptance" as the act of decreasing maladaptive struggles to change one's partner's behavior, and using discussion of problems and differences as a way to achieve greater closeness. It is important to note that the purpose of acceptance is not to encourage couples to ignore problems, be resigned to their current level of relationship satisfaction, or accept the status quo. Rather, it is designed to help couples use their differences as vehicles to achieve greater intimacy and thereby improve their relationship. For those couples who have difficulty collaborating or changing their behavior, acceptance offers a viable alternative approach to building a closer relationship. For couples who do benefit from the more traditional, change-oriented approach, emotional acceptance interventions can enhance their progress, because most couples have some problems that seem impervious to change. Furthermore, one of the paradoxes of acceptance work is that it may actually facilitate behavior change more effectively than traditional change strategies. The goal of emotional acceptance is to reduce partners' maladaptive struggles to change one another, especially because the pressure to change may, in some cases, prevent change from occurring (Jacobson, Christensen, Prince, Cordova, & Eldridge, 2000).

Three broad categories of interventions in IBCT are designed to promote emotional acceptance. *Empathic joining* encourages the expression of thoughts and feelings that are likely to meet with empathy and understanding, rather than defensiveness, anger, or invalidation, from one's partner. For example, the therapist may solicit the expression of "softer" emotions (sadness, hurt, loneliness) rather than "harder" emotions (anger or resentment). In another empathic joining intervention, the therapist may reformulate a partner's behavior, emphasizing his or her efforts, however misdirected, to address a problem, or may remind one partner of the historical or contextual factors that help to make sense of and increase a sympathetic perspective toward the other partner's problematic behavior. *Unified detachment* encourages partners to engage in an intellectual analysis of their problems and to view problems as outside of themselves. In discussions promoting unified detachment, the therapist is careful to avoid or reframe any evaluative statements that place blame or responsibility for change on one person. The goal is to reframe the problem not as "mine" or "yours," but as an "it," a common adversary with which partners need to cope together. This is done through a variety of techniques, including learning to debrief arguments to identify the usual sequence of events that leads to problematic incidents, increasing awareness of the continuity between various incidents, and developing insight into the relationship between incidents and core themes in the relationship. Humor and metaphor can also be used to promote a detached, nonblaming analysis of the problem. Finally, *tolerance building* is designed to promote emotional acceptance by increasing a spouse's tolerance for his or her partner's problematic behavior. This is accomplished through highlighting the positive features of negative behavior, "faking" incidents of negative behavior to promote desensitization to inevitable slip ups, and increasing self-care in the face of negative partner behavior. The rationale behind these strategies is that even when positive change is accomplished as a result of therapy, instances of negative behavior inevitably occur; if partners can decrease their vulnerability to each other's problem behaviors and to inevitable conflicts, greater intimacy can be achieved.

In IBCT, acceptance strategies are integrated with the change-oriented strategies of TBCT. The relative emphasis on acceptance versus change depends on the couple's clinical presentation, their individual and relationship characteristics, and the therapist's assessment of their ability to collaborate. The integration of change and acceptance strategies is covered further when we discuss assessment and case conceptualization, and is illustrated when we return to the case examples later in this chapter. Cordova (2002) proposes that this integrative approach, which emphasizes a functional analysis of each couple's interactions and problematic behaviors, allows more flexibility and is better equipped to deal with the wide variety of clinical issues presented in therapy.

In initial studies, IBCT has shown considerable promise in overcoming some of the limitations of TBCT. In one study, the in-session interactions of couples treated with IBCT began to change over the course of therapy, with partners engaging in more expression of "soft" emotion and decreased blaming of one another (Cordova, Jacobson, & Christensen, 1998). Furthermore, in a small pilot study, Jacobson et al. (2000) found that both husbands and wives treated with IBCT reported greater increases in marital satisfaction than those treated with TBCT. It was hoped that IBCT would both reach those couples for whom collaboration is more difficult and increase the durability of gains made during therapy. Currently, a large, multisite trial comparing IBCT with TBCT is under way. This study will provide a more definitive test of the efficacy and durability of IBCT. To date, however, no studies of TBCT or IBCT have included same-sex couples; this would be an important addition to the literature on treatment of relationship discord.

COGNITIVE-BEHAVIORAL THERAPY FOR COUPLES: MODIFYING DYSFUNCTIONAL BELIEFS AND EXPECTATIONS

CBT for couples (Baucom & Epstein, 1990; Beck, 1988; Dattilio & Padesky, 1990) is similar to TBCT in that it places importance on the role of environmental influences on partner behavior. However, CBT adds an emphasis on intrapersonal factors, and, in particular, on cognition. Following directly from CBT for individuals, a central tenet of CBT for couples is that cognition mediates the relationship between environment and behavior. So, for example, an individual whose partner forgets an important anniversary may conclude that his partner doesn't care, or he may attribute his partner's lapse to being overwhelmed with a work project deadline. These two different attributions would in turn result in very different emotional reactions and behavioral responses, which would evoke different responses in the second partner, and so on. In CBT, couples learn to look for and examine their dysfunctional or inaccurate perceptions, attributions, and expectations regarding the partner and relationships in general. Couples therefore learn to be careful of automatically accepting their first interpretation of a partner's behavior or a situation, especially if they are upset, when interpretations are most likely to be extreme and problematic. Cognitions are evaluated in terms of not only their validity but also their impact on the relationship. For example, an individual who believes that all of her emotional needs should be met by her partner might be asked to examine the pros and cons of holding this belief, and the effect it has had on her relationship satisfaction and behavior. Couples not only gain insight into how their dysfunctional cognitions and the concomitant behaviors are contributing to relationship discord but also learn how to modify their thoughts and constructions of reality. This is accomplished through a number of techniques similar to those used in individual CBT, including checking one's perceptions with the other person, gathering evidence to test cognitions, and examining the costs and benefits of particular cognitions. CBT for couples integrates cognitive interventions with the behavior change strategies of TBCT, using behavior exchange, communication training, and problem-solving training to target problematic relationship behaviors.

The cognitive model of relationship distress assumes that cognitions, feelings, and behavior are all interdependent; therefore, intervention in one domain is likely to produce change in other domains. For example, a partner who begins to learn skills to clearly communicate his needs might change the dysfunctional belief that his partner should be able to intuit his needs at all times. Conversely, a particular problematic behavior (or the absence of a positive behavior) may be related to beliefs and expectations rather than to a skills deficit per se. For example, an individual who does not ask for time alone from her partner may avoid doing so, not because this skill is lacking in her behavioral repertoire, but because she believes it is unacceptable to do so. In this case, simply targeting the behavior is unlikely to be effective, whereas targeting the cognition may lead to behavior change.

In an early study, couples treated with cognitive interventions in addition to TBCT had better outcomes than minimal treatment controls (Margolin & Weiss, 1978), although studies directly comparing cognitive strategies to traditional behavioral couple therapy have yielded mixed results (Baucom & Epstein, 1990). Although CBT for gay and lesbian couples has not been empirically validated, Dattilio and Padesky (1990) briefly discuss its application to same-sex couples. They suggest that issues frequently faced by same-sex couples, including social isolation and lack of support, negative beliefs about the self, and increased stress related to the AIDS epidemic, can be addressed effectively by CBT. As with IBCT, a clinical outcome study including same-sex couples would be an important addition to the literature.

ASSESSMENT AND CASE CONCEPTUALIZATION

A thorough assessment and clear case conceptualization are critical to effective couple therapy. In their discussion of IBCT, Christensen, Jacobson, and Babcock (1995) suggest a four-session format for initial assessment. Although suggested by the proponents of IBCT, this format would lend itself well to CBT. The couple is first seen for an initial, conjoint session. The primary goals of the initial session are to establish rapport with the couple; to assess for imminent crises (e.g., suicidal or homicidal ideation, psychosis symptoms, domestic violence); to refer the couple for immediate intervention, if necessary; to gather information about the relationship history and current problems; to begin to formulate tentative hypotheses and treatment goals; and to instill hope that therapy can help. Couples are given self-report questionnaires to complete at home (we suggest some self-report measures shortly).

Next, each partner is seen for one individual session, during which the clinician gathers information regarding the individual's psychosocial and psychiatric history. This session also provides each partner with an opportunity to disclose important and sensitive topics such as affairs, domestic violence, sexual dysfunction, child abuse, or steps taken toward separation or divorce about which the other partner may not yet know. It is important to establish with the couple beforehand how secrets divulged during individual sessions will be handled. The most common approach is to remind couples beforehand that anything divulged in an individual session may be brought up in subsequent conjoint sessions based on the therapist's best judgment. Some therapists recommend giving couples a choice of "secrets policies": They can choose either the traditional, "no secrets" approach, or to have the therapist hold confidences, but only if both partners agree (e.g., Spring, 2001). It is felt that the latter option allows the therapist to press for the truth regarding controversial issues such as affairs. However, a recent study has indicated that couples in which an affair took place and was not revealed during therapy were more distressed and had poorer treatment outcomes than couples with affairs that were discussed in therapy (Atkins, 2002).

Self-Report Questionnaires

Several self-report questionnaires are mentioned here that can be helpful additions to clinical interview. Unfortunately, the vast majority of these measures have been normed on heterosexual couples and are written in heterosexist language, such as using gender-specific pronouns, and references to "husband" and "wife" and to marriage and divorce. These measures can all be easily modified to be gender nonspecific, however, and refer to "relationships" and "partners." However, comparison with norms established on heterosexual samples is tentative at best until these measures are normed on same-sex couples.

Domains of Relationship Assessment

During the initial conjoint and individual sessions, therapists can organize their thinking around the following six questions (Christensen et al., 1995):

How Distressed Is This Couple?

Level of relationship distress is often quite apparent in the initial interview. How overtly angry are the partners with each other? Can they listen to one another without yelling, interrupting, or blaming? On the other hand, do they seem emotionally disengaged? Have they separated or discussed separation? Self-report measures of distress can provide additional, quantitative data regarding distress, as well as a baseline to compare with posttherapy levels of distress. For example, the Dyadic Adjustment Scale (DAS; Spanier, 1976), a widely used measure of relationship satisfaction, has good construct validity and reliability, and is written in gender-neutral language. Regardless of level of distress, relationship violence should also be assessed. This can be done through an interview, but it is also helpful to supplement interview indications with a self-report questionnaire such as the Conflict Tactics Scale (CTS; Straus, 1979; Straus, Hamby, Boney-McCoy, & Sugarman, 1996). The individual session then provides an excellent opportunity to follow up on any indications of significant violence from this questionnaire. The CTS is written in gender-neutral language.

How Committed Is the Couple to the Relationship and to Treatment?

A couple's level of commitment to the relationship, despite the problems they may be experiencing, is an important prognostic indicator for treatment, because it speaks to how willing partners may be to put in the effort required by therapy. For many couples, commitment diminishes as level of relationship distress increases, but it is important not to assume that commitment and distress are always inversely related. For example, a couple might be very volatile and distressed about the relationship, yet be highly committed; this couple may actually be more likely to benefit from therapy than a couple that is extremely disengaged and therefore not reporting much conflict or distress. An excellent self-report measure of commitment is the Marital Status Inventory (MSI; Weiss & Cerreto, 1980), which asks couples to check off items reflecting thoughts of and steps taken toward separation, with more steps taken indicating lower commitment to the relationship. The MSI is written for heterosexual couples, with gender-specific language and references to "marriage" and "divorce," but can easily be revised for same-sex couples.

Another indication of commitment is each partner's capacity for change and accommodation to his or her partner. Whereas some partners seem predisposed toward compromise, others may say that they have done all that they can or maintain that only the partner needs to change. Some questions to ask to ascertain capacity for collaboration include "How do you contribute to the problems in your relationship (or to a particular problem)?" and "What are some of the changes that you could make to improve your relationship?" Individuals who can pinpoint specific things they could do differently (apart from just increasing their tolerance of their partner's negative behavior) may be more committed to the relationship and to the therapy process than those who cannot.

Although level of commitment can be ascertained from the initial conjoint session and self-report questionnaires, it may be most apparent in individual sessions. For example, one or both partners may reveal that they have already given up on the relationship and see therapy as a "last resort." Some individuals come to couple therapy, whether consciously or not, to provide safety and support for their partner while they separate. Or one or both partners may reveal affairs that severely limit commitment to the relationship. Level of commitment provides the therapist with important information regarding the couple's resources available for therapy and also informs the choice of initial treatment interventions. To the extent that commitment is very low, couples are less likely to be able to accommodate and compromise; for these couples, emotional acceptance interventions may be a better place to start than change strategies.

What Issues Divide the Couple?

Most couples can readily discuss their areas of disagreement during initial interviews, and self-report inventories can further reveal areas of disagreement that partners may not think of or may be reluctant to bring up during the initial therapy session. The first section of the DAS lists several areas about which couples often disagree, assessing level of conflict about each. The Who Does What Questionnaire (Cowan, Cowan, Coie, & Coie, 1978) assesses partners' perceptions of their relative responsibility for household tasks, child care, and decision making, and gives an indication of problems specific to division of labor. The original measure is written with gender-specific pronouns, but it can be easily modified for use with same-sex couples. Another useful self-report measure is the Frequency and Acceptability of Partner Behavior (Christensen & Jacobson, 1997; Doss & Christensen, 1999), which asks respondents to rate both the frequency of a variety of positive and negative partner behaviors, and the acceptability of those behaviors at their current frequency. This gender-neutral questionnaire can give the clinician important information about partners' perceptions of one another's behavior, as well as the contribution of specific behaviors to the individual's relationship distress. The full questionnaire is reproduced in Appendix II. This measure can help the clinician avoid making incorrect assumptions regarding the relative importance of various relationship issues. Even seemingly trivial behaviors, because of factors such as the couple's learning history or what that particular behavior represents to the individual, may be highly distressing, whereas other behaviors that might seem quite problematic may not be so for a particular couple. For example, although sexual non-monogamy is acceptable to some gay male couples, it may be highly distressing to a heterosexual couple. Conversely, a seemingly trivial behavior, such as not doing the dishes, can take on very significant meaning for a distressed couple that has a great deal of conflict over division of labor. It is also important to elucidate not only the problem areas, but also each partner's position on the issue. For example, a couple's endorsement of money as an area of disagreement could mean many things. One partner may be referring to different spending styles and approaches to saving, whereas the other may be feeling resentful about being the primary earner in the family. Individual sessions provide an excellent opportunity to follow up on areas of conflict indicated on self-report questionnaires, and to elucidate each partner's position on topics endorsed as problems.

Why Are These Issues Such a Problem for the Couple?

Whereas the previous question related to the *content* of disagreements, this one relates to the *process* by which couples try to deal with their disagreements. It is often the process, including the couple's maladaptive efforts to solve relationship problems, that is causing considerable distress. Couples often mention deficits in their communication and problem-solving abilities. For example, a client may feel that her partner doesn't listen well, or that problems never get solved because conflict discussions get so heated that both partners withdraw before solutions have been entertained. Furthermore, the couple may engage in particular interaction patterns that inevitably lead to conflict. Christensen et al. (1995) highlight three such interaction patterns. In *mutual traps*, partners' well-intentioned efforts to solve the problem result in the very behavior in their partner that they don't want. One very common mutual trap is seen in couples struggling with differences in desired level of closeness, resulting in a "demand–withdrawal" interaction pattern (Christensen, 1987; Christensen & Heavey, 1990; Jacobson, 1989). One partner, dissatisfied with the current level of intimacy, presses his or her partner for more closeness through requests, complaints, or criticisms. The other partner, comfortable with the status quo or wanting more independence, resists change by maintaining or increasing distance. This mutual trap is associated with relationship distress for partners in both roles. A second interaction pattern is *minefields*, "hot buttons" that virtually always lead to severe conflict. For some couples, money may be a minefield; for others, the relationship with in-laws. Regardless of the content, a minefield has great significance for the couple, inevitably leads to extreme conflict, may be avoided, and never gets resolved. Finally, a *credibility gap* refers to an impasse reached because one partner's position in an argument is simply not believable to the other partner: for example, when one partner insists that he or she wants the other to change eating habits, out of concern for the other's health, while he or she engages in obviously un-healthy behaviors (e.g., smoking, not exercising). The lack of credibility makes problem solving difficult or impossible, because partners do not start with a shared view of the problem. For a therapist taking a cogni-tive approach, this domain also includes assessment of partners' percep-tions and cognitions that may be impacting relationship satisfaction. For example, the Relationship Belief Inventory (RBI; Eidelson & Ep-stein, 1982) assesses each partner's relationship beliefs and standards, and can form the basis for an examination of beliefs and assumptions that may be contributing to relationship distress.

What Are the Couple's Strengths?

Another way to frame this question is to ask couples what is keeping them together, despite the problems they are having. Some individuals may readily be able to identify their strengths as a couple and qualities of their partner that they continue to find reinforcing. For others, this may be much more difficult; for these couples, it is often helpful to ask partners what attracted them to one another in the first place. It is inter-esting to note that, often, the very qualities that attracted partners to one another initially are identified as problematic now. This part of the assessment can therefore lay the groundwork for later reformulation of problematic behaviors in a more favorable light. Another question to ask is how they have dealt with hard times; a couple who is very dis-tressed may nonetheless have great resilience and may have dealt with major stressors together, giving the partners a strong sense of unity. Finally, it is helpful to assess a couple's idiosyncratic repair strategies. For example, many couples use humor to reduce tension and move to-ward repair after an argument. It is much more beneficial to identify and build on existing success strategies than to use rules from commu-nication manuals to help couples move through conflict.

How Can Therapy Help?

This question is answered by developing a treatment plan that might in-clude determining whether initial emphasis will be on change or accep-tance strategies, what skills deficits will be addressed, the particular content areas that should receive attention, and so on. Although the treatment plan does not need to be written out, we have found it helpful to write out the plan, as well as the answers to the previous five assessment questions, so that they can be referred to throughout treatment. Sample treatment plans for the two couples presented in this chapter follow in a later section, after we have provided additional case material.

In developing the treatment plan, it is also helpful to take into account the couple's baseline functioning and realistically appraise how much improvement can be expected. Clearly, the prognosis is different for extremely distressed or extremely disengaged couples, or for those who have already made plans to separate or are separated. The couple's value system and individual partners' functioning may also impact the amount of improvement that can realistically be expected. For example, a couple in which one partner has a significant psychiatric disorder may have a less favorable prognosis than a couple not facing these problems.

Feedback Session

The partners are again seen together during the fourth session. During this "feedback session," information gathered from the previous three sessions, as well as from self-report questionnaires, is integrated into a case conceptualization that is presented to the couple, and the partners agree on a treatment plan. The six questions can be used as an outline to present information to the couple, with feedback regarding their level of relationship distress and commitment, key content areas of disagreement, problematic interaction patterns and cognitions, strengths, and an initial outline of how therapy can help. Although a large amount of information is presented to the couple during this session, it is not meant to be a lecture by the therapist, but is rather an interactive process between the therapist and the couple, with the therapist presenting tentative hypotheses, asking the couple for their feedback, and continuing to refine the case conceptualization. Self-report data can be utilized here in multiple ways. For example, scores on paper-and-pencil measures may be used to reassure a highly anxious couple, or to underscore the seriousness of the situation to partners who are minimizing their problems. Couples can also be reminded that self-report questionnaires can be readministered at the end of therapy, providing an objective measure of treatment progress. Appendix III provides a summary sheet for therapists who prefer to have clients take notes in the session. This allows the couple to have a written summary of several of the points discussed in the feedback session.

Finally, the feedback session marks the beginning of the intervention phase of treatment, as well as the end of formal assessment. For example, during delineation of a couple's strengths, the therapist can begin to reformulate some problems related to the very qualities that attracted them to one another in the first place. An individual who complains about his partner's inability to plan may be reminded that his partner's spontaneity was a quality that drew him initially (if, in fact, this is the case). Another type of intervention that takes place during the feedback session is to challenge partners with very low commitment to assess whether they are willing to put forth the effort required by therapy. The therapist can emphasize the fact that the success of therapy depends in large part on their efforts, and that no matter how skilled the therapist, treatment is only beneficial with a couple that wants an improved relationship. In general, the feedback session serves two purposes: it both provides the couple with a descriptive framework for understanding their problems and begins to move them in a positive direction in terms of viewing their problems as shared and enhancing hopefulness about their ability to improve their relationship.

TREATMENT PLANNING: WHAT TO DO FIRST?

Several factors go into treatment planning in cognitive and behavioral couple therapy approaches, including the case conceptualization and the couple's current level of distress, commitment, and potential for collaboration. In TBCT, treatment typically begins with behavior exchange strategies to increase the couple's frequency of positive interactions and thereby increase motivation for treatment. Treatment typically then moves into communication training and problem-solving training. In problem-solving training, couples practice on their actual problems identified in the initial assessment and/or that come up as therapy proceeds. Generally, couples are asked to focus first on smaller, less emotionally intense issues; as their skills increase, they can be applied to more substantive areas of concern. The final stages of treatment in TBCT focus on generalization of skills and strategies to maintain gains and prevent relapse.

In IBCT, the couple's level of distress and the degree to which partners can collaborate and take shared responsibility for their problems inform which types of interventions are initially emphasized. For example, for some couples who are mildly to moderately distressed and highly collaborative, change strategies such as behavior exchange, communication, and problem solving may be introduced first. However, even for these couples, acceptance strategies may be utilized to enhance closeness and pave the way for change. For example, even in couples who are willing to collaborate, individuals may need to increase their understanding of and "soften" their position toward the partner's negative behavior before problem solving can be undertaken. For couples who are highly distressed and/or have little capacity for collaboration, it is often beneficial to begin with acceptance-based interventions. Rather than encouraging the individuals to continue to blame one another by focusing on the partner's need for change, acceptance interventions are more likely to promote tolerance and understanding of one another's negative behaviors, and may increase feelings of closeness in spite of serious relationship problems.

In cognitive-behavioral couple therapy, the therapist takes a pragmatic and individualized approach to choosing initial interventions, focusing on the domain that seems most likely to result in early success as an initial target (Chapman & Dehle, 2002). For example, for some couples, it may be easier to learn new receptive and expressive communication skills than to focus on dysfunctional relationship beliefs or expectations; for these couples, communication training might be undertaken first. Because the cognitive model of relationship distress assumes that cognitions, behaviors, and feelings are all interrelated, the therapist is free to choose any of the three domains as an initial focus of treatment.

Gary and Walter: Emotional Acceptance Leads to Behavior Change

The level of distress Gary and Walter were experiencing was apparent even as they sat in the waiting room prior to their first therapy session. They sat far apart on the couch, making no conversation and no eye contact. During the session, they related the relationship history presented at the beginning of this chapter. The therapist noted that while one was talking, the other frequently gave nonverbal indications of disagreement or even contempt (shaking his head, sighing, rolling his eyes). Also, the therapist noted that Walter frequently interrupted when Gary was talking.

Their self-report measures and individual sessions further confirmed their level of distress and emotional disengagement. Whereas Gary scored a 96 on the DAS, close to the established cutoff of 97 for separating distressed from nondistressed couples, Walter scored a 75, well below the cutoff and indicating significant distress. On the MSI, both indicated having had many thoughts of separation and talking to friends about the possibility of separation. In fact, they had separated already to some degree by moving into separate bedrooms. Walter, in particular, seemed to have disengaged considerably; during his individual interview, he revealed feeling quite hopeless about the relationship and stated that therapy was a "last-ditch effort" to save the relationship.

A primary issue identified by both as problematic was their communication skills. Gary accused Walter of frequently "shutting down" during discussion of conflictual topics. Problems rarely got solved, because once Gary started yelling, Walter would usually leave the room or the house, and neither would return to the discussion later. Both indicated that Gary's emotions frequently escalated during arguments, with dramatic or provocative statements such as threatening to leave the relationship or saying that his life would be over without Walter.

Another issue that became clear during assessment was that the couple had differences in their desired level of closeness, with Gary wanting more togetherness and a more exclusive relationship, and Walter desiring more independence. Furthermore, Walter was uncomfortable with what he perceived as Gary's level of dependence on him, and said that he often felt "smothered" by Gary. He wanted Gary to have more social outlets apart from their relationship, and to gain more financial independence. On Gary's part, he wanted Walter to be able to confide in him more, communicate about his feelings, and express both verbal and nonverbal affection.

When asked about their strengths, both partners had some difficulty answering. Both identified their history, including 10 years together, as well as owning a home and several pets together, as things that bonded them. Gary said that he still felt very attracted to Walter, and that Walter was a "genuinely nice person underneath all the gruffness."

During the feedback session, the therapist presented information to Gary and Walter regarding their level of distress and commitment, and highlighted content issues that seemed most salient, including the question of monogamy. The therapist also discussed process issues, focusing particularly on their differences in desired level of closeness and "demand–withdrawal" interaction pattern, also using the feedback session as an opportunity to challenge Walter regarding his apparent low level of commitment and disengagement from the relationship by asking him whether he felt able to put forth the effort required by therapy; in a sense, the therapist asked Walter for some indication that therapy was going to be a worthwhile endeavor. Walter noted that in the weeks since beginning treatment, there had been some improvement in their relationship, with less yelling and more "kindness" toward each other; he thought that both felt relieved that they were finally getting some help, and the slight improvement they'd experienced gave him increased hope and motivation for treatment.

In deciding on initial treatment strategies, the therapist noted that Walter and Gary were quite distressed and disengaged, that they were polarized in terms of not only their relative resources and power (Walter was significantly older, had a more prestigious job, made more money, and owned their home) but also their views of a healthy relationship, with Gary valuing closeness and exclusivity more than Walter. Given these factors, the therapist decided to begin with IBCT acceptance strategies and planned to move to traditional change strategies and skills building as their positions toward one another softened. The initial treatment plan for Gary and Walter is provided in Table 6.1.

TABLE 6.1. Treatment Plan for Gary and Walter

Problem	Intervention
Emotional disengagement and polarization	Emotional acceptance strategies • Debrief recent problem interactions • Empathic joining • Elicit "soft" emotions • Encourage unified detachment (seeing problem as "it")
Communication deficits • Criticalness, escalation, diverting to other topics (Gary) • Stonewalling (Walter)	Teach communication skills; practice in session and at home • "I" statements • Active listening • Paraphrasing
Lack of conflict resolution skills	Teach problem-solving skills; practice in session and at home
Conflicts over amount of closeness versus independence; "pursuing–distancing" interaction pattern	• Explain "mutual trap" • Debrief typical interactions; encourage empathic joining, unified detachment, and self-care in face of negative behavior • Use communication and problem-solving skills to negotiate amount of time spent together
Conflict regarding monogamy	• Use emotional acceptance techniques to relate issue to core conflict over closeness–independence • Use communication and problem-solving skills to negotiate acceptable solution
Generalization and maintenance	• Reduce therapist prompts • Homework assignments • "State of the relationship" meetings

The therapist focused initially on Walter and Gary's differences in desired level of closeness, engaging the couple in discussions designed to encourage their empathic joining around the problem. For example, as noted earlier, Walter often withdrew during discussion of conflictual topics, and this would anger Gary. The therapist asked Gary whether he was feeling other emotions during those times besides anger. Gary was able to identify feelings of hurt, loneliness, and fear that Walter would leave him. Gary's learning history was explored for experiences that might have made him especially sensitive to Walter's withdrawal. He related a history of having felt rejected by many people in his life: He was often teased in school and also felt rejected by his father, who left the family and never recontacted the children after divorcing their mother. He felt that Walter was "the only person who had ever really been there for him." Gary really did fear being abandoned by Walter and wasn't just making such statements to be provocative; as Gary found less provocative ways to talk about his fears, Walter was more able to hear him. The therapist also elicited from Walter aspects of his family of origin that seemed relevant to his role in the problem. Walter came from a family in which his father was cold, remote, and occasionally physically abusive toward his mother. This background not only provided Walter with very little modeling of relationship intimacy but also caused him to be avoidant of conflict, because he never wanted to be abusive like his father. Their disclosure of more vulnerable emotions and historical context helped Walter and Gary to feel more sympathetic toward one another's positions.

Interventions also focused on promoting a stance of unified detachment toward their problems. For example, the therapist encouraged them to "debrief" recent arguments, describing in great detail the events leading up to and during an argument. As they reviewed several incidents, Walter and Gary began to clearly see the pattern their conflicts usually followed. Gary would often bring up an issue that was bothering him when Walter was already somewhat distracted, for example, when reading the newspaper or watching the news. As Gary grew more frustrated and pursued Walter's attention further, Walter would disengage more, doing what Gary described as "shutting down." This would upset and anger Gary, leading to his escalating the argument with yelling and threats. Eventually, Walter would walk away from the situation or leave the house. Both began to see this pattern as a "mutual trap," in which each partner's behavior elicited exactly the behavior he didn't want in the other partner. They began to see the problem as something they did together, their "dance," and would sometimes come in to a session laughing, saying, "Well, we did it again."

The initial focus on emotional acceptance resulted in Walter and Gary softening their positions toward one another and feeling closer despite no change having occurred in their presenting problems. Having accomplished this, they were more willing to collaborate and focus on behavior change, and in the next phase of therapy they began to practice communication and problem-solving skills. Each learned to use "I statements," focusing on his own feelings rather than blaming his partner, and learned a structured format for solving problems. As is often the case, their deficits in communication skills were functionally related to the "core" topics that were problematic for them. For example, Walter's communication style was related to the couple's struggles with power and independence. Although Walter said he wanted an equal relationship with Gary and didn't want to be a "father figure," he exerted his power in various ways in the relationship, for example, by frequently interrupting when Gary was speaking. The therapist pointed this out to him in the session and encouraged him to work on listening until Gary was finished and using "active listening" skills to let Gary know he'd been heard and understood. This helped Gary feel less "dominated" conversationally and also opened the door to discussion of other ways in which Walter dominated Gary, despite his stated desire that Gary become more independent. In this way, traditional skills building and emotional acceptance work proceeded together rather than serially.

One important content area and focus of therapy was the issue of non-monogamy. The therapist was aware that a unique norm of gay male relationships is that sex outside of the primary relationship can for some couples be an accepted part of the relationship (this is discussed further in an earlier section of this chapter). While not pathologizing the couple's interest in non-monogamy, it was important to look at the function non-monogamy might be serving in their relationship. In Walter and Gary's case, Walter had pursued an outside relationship at a time when he was feeling very "smothered" by Gary's dependence on him, as a way to distance himself further from Gary. On his part, Gary revealed that it wasn't Walter having sex with other men per se that had upset him, but Walter's deception and secrecy in seeking out this other relationship. Once these issues were discussed, they could more clearly explore their wishes with regard to non-monogamy. This discussion revealed that Walter was more interested in sexual non-monogamy than Gary, but Gary was comfortable consenting to Walter having outside experiences as long as he disclosed them. They eventually agreed on the following: They would continue to consider themselves to be "emotionally monogamous," but sex outside of the relationship was acceptable; any encounters by either partner would be "recreational" only, and each would tell the other about any outside experiences.

As therapy progressed, some unexpected changes occurred that had not been targeted directly by the therapist's interventions. As Gary began to acknowledge to himself, and to Walter, his fears of abandonment and low sense of self-reliance, he began to do some work on his own. He participated in workshops to increase his eligibility for a job promotion, and he began to spend some time with his own set of friends. He also came to therapy one night, stating that he had conducted a financial analysis and realized that he could survive financially without Walter if he needed to, although it would mean living more modestly. Gary realized, and communicated to Walter, that he would survive if their relationship broke up, both financially and emotionally. Not only did Gary feel more confident but also Walter felt less pressured and said he felt that now he could decide to stay in the relationship because he wanted to, not because he was afraid Gary wouldn't survive without him. Prior to emotional acceptance work, both partners had been too rigid in their positions and too disillusioned with one another to entertain mutual requests for change. Now Gary was making some of the changes that, at the onset of therapy, Walter had been asking for but Gary had been unwilling or unable to make. This session turned out to be pivotal to the couple's progress. Shortly after, their sessions tapered to every other week and focused on helping them generalize the changes they had made and discuss ways to maintain improvement after therapy ended. They committed to bimonthly "state of the relationship" meetings, during which they agreed that they would discuss any issues that had come up since the last meeting and work on conflict resolution. After four sessions focused on generalization and maintenance, the couple terminated. Their final interview and repeated self-report measures revealed that their relationship satisfaction and commitment to one another had improved.

Julia and Ellie: Modifying Dysfunctional Relationship Beliefs

When Julia and Ellie came to therapy, they described themselves as being in a second "honeymoon" phase, having just gotten back together after their 2-month separation. Both partners scored in the nondistressed range on the DAS and indicated a high degree of commitment to the relationship, but they said that the picture would have been very different had they answered questionnaires a few months earlier. Both felt that they had many good relationship "tools" already; for example, they felt skilled in communication and able to discuss difficult topics. However, they did not fully understand the events that had led to their separation and felt a sense of unease that the same thing could happen again.

In conducting the assessment with Julia and Ellie, the therapist noted that this was the first long-term lesbian relationship for both women, and considered it important to assess their beliefs about lesbian relationships. The therapist discovered that Ellie, who had recently divorced, had many idealized beliefs about lesbian relationships, including that they would be much closer than heterosexual ones, that two women together would "understand each other all the time," and that she would not experience the same level of conflict she had with her husband. Julia, on the other hand, held some negative beliefs about the viability of same-sex partnerships. She thought that they "never lasted," and that there usually wasn't the same level of commitment as in heterosexual relationships. Neither woman could identify any positive role models for long-term, committed same-sex relationships, in part because they had few gay and lesbian friends.

In this case, the therapist decided to proceed with a cognitive approach. Both partners already possessed good communication skills. Also, given their low level of distress and high degree of commitment, the prognosis for collaboration was good for them. The case conceptualization for this couple focused primarily on their unrealistic expectations regarding relationships, which seemed to contribute to relationship distress and problematic behavior. Table 6.2 presents the treatment plan for Julia and Ellie.

In the early sessions of therapy, Julia and Ellie were presented with the cognitive-behavioral model of relationship distress, which empha-

TABLE 6.2. Treatment Plan for Julia and Ellie

Problem	Intervention
Unrealistic beliefs regarding lesbian relationships	• Modify unrealistic beliefs • Behavioral experiments
Negative attributions regarding partner's behavior	• Gather evidence • Consider pros and cons of attributions • Generate alternative attributions
Conflicts over amount of closeness versus independence	• Explore relationship expectations • Psychoeducation regarding normative development of lesbian relationships • Use of communication and problem-solving skills to generate acceptable solutions
Lack of social support and positive role models	• Increase contact and friendship with other gay/lesbian couples • Provide information regarding community resources
Generalization and maintenance	• Reduce therapist prompts • Homework assignments • "State of the relationship" meetings

sizes the interplay among cognitive, affective, and behavioral aspects of experience. The model was rooted in examples from their own history to help them understand it as well as to develop a common conceptual framework within which to view their relationship problems. For example, the therapist pointed out that, in her marriage, Ellie had often felt misunderstood by her husband, yet she felt very understood and validated by her female friends. These environmental factors led to her belief that Julia should know what she needed all the time, without Ellie having to tell her. This led to a problematic behavior, Ellie not voicing her needs, that in turn led to Julia sometimes not knowing and responding to her needs. When this occurred, Ellie tended to feel let down, disappointed, and angry.

Once Julia and Ellie had a good grasp of the model, the therapist began encouraging them to challenge some of their unrealistic expectations, for example, asking Ellie to consider whether it was reasonable to expect Julia to "mind read," and whether Ellie herself always knew what Julia needed. Also, the therapist emphasized that, given the interrelatedness of cognition, affect, and behavior, this meant that the couple could intervene in any of these domains. Ellie could work on changing her expectation, which might lead to different behavior (voicing her needs); alternatively, she could change the behavior, which might lead to different consequences (getting her needs met more often) and affect (more relationship satisfaction). Ellie was not being assertive about her needs, not because she didn't possess this skill, but because she believed that she didn't need to do so with a female partner. The behavior of assertion was already in her repertoire, and once the cognition began to change, so did the behavior: Ellie began to assert her needs more frequently. A positive environmental response (Julia listening to her, and trying to meet her needs) reinforced both the cognitive and the behavioral changes.

A similar pattern was seen with regard to Ellie's and Julia's expectations about getting needs met within versus outside of the relationship. Ellie again acknowledged having a somewhat idealized view of the lesbian relationship, in which she thought that most of her needs would be met. Julia, who had been single for some time before getting together with Ellie, valued her time alone and liked to pursue various leisure activities, spend time with friends, or just "decompress." Ellie tended to interpret Julia's desire for separateness as a statement that she didn't care for her as much as she had in the beginning of their relationship. Ellie was asked to consider the pros and cons of this attribution, and to gather evidence for and against her attribution about Julia's behavior. For example, she noted that Julia was the one who had ended their separation and had suggested couple therapy, a strong indicator of her commitment and caring. Ellie was helped to generate alternative attributions that had more pros and fewer cons. She was able to come up with several alternative attributions, including the fact that Julia used physical exercise to help her unwind from work, and that there were interests Julia shared with other friends, such as working on art projects, that she didn't share with Ellie. A psychoeducational approach was also useful in helping Ellie to develop more realistic expectations; in session, she was provided with information and reading material about the normative development of lesbian relationships, including information concerning lesbians' tendency to need to build healthy independence into their relationship (e.g., Clunis & Green, 2000).

It was also important to validate the aspects of Ellie's perceptions that were accurate. As therapy progressed, Julia was able to acknowledge that she had begun to feel stifled in the relationship, and that "picking fights," decreased sexual contact, and finally moving out were all attempts to increase distance between them when she felt unable to do so in a healthy way within the relationship. The couple began to recognize and were relieved to have insight into the pattern that had led to the separation. Julia began to feel that it was acceptable to ask for some separateness, and that doing so would not be as upsetting to Ellie.

Although Ellie's unrealistically positive relationship expectations had contributed to their earlier problems and were the primary focus at the beginning of therapy, Julia's negative relationship beliefs also had an impact. She held several negative beliefs regarding the viability of same-sex relationships, including "They never last," "They're all about sex," and "Gay couples don't know how to commit." When asked where she'd first heard these opinions, she said that she had heard them in her family; she noted that she had a cousin, her only gay relative, in his 20s, whose mother (Julia's aunt) frequently complained to Julia's mother about his "lifestyle." Her family's homophobia was further evidenced in her mother's negative response regarding the possibility of a lesbian couple having children. Julia had internalized these beliefs, which were further exacerbated by her virtual lack of social support and few models for healthy same-sex relationships. To address this, Julia and Ellie were given a behavioral "homework assignment" to make connections with some gay and lesbian friends in general, and couples in particular. Both were still uncomfortable coming out at work, so they decided to pursue friendships through outside activities. Together, they joined a lesbian choral group, and Julia joined a gay and lesbian running club that met weekly for jogs around the city. Through these groups, they began to make friends, and, at one point, were invited to the commitment ceremony of a lesbian couple (in their chorus) that had already been together for several years. They also met several gay and lesbian parents.

These experiences not only helped Julia to challenge some of her negative beliefs but also exposed the couple to an array of choices in terms of creating family, community, and tradition. They began to take some steps of their own toward greater commitment; for example, they enlisted the services of a gay attorney to draw up health care power of attorney, specifying that they could make important medical decisions for each other, and they began to look into buying a house together.

At termination, Julia and Ellie reported much increased awareness into the problems that had led to their separation, and increased confidence that they could make their relationship work. They continued to work on finding a balance between time spent together and time apart, and devised some creative ways to build this into their relationship; for example, one weeknight every week was marked as "girls' night out," during which it was understood that either or both of them would go out with separate friends. They continued to have occasional disagreements but found that many of their arguments were caused by one of them having expectations or needs she wasn't voicing; both felt that they were able to repair these conflicts much more easily. They had begun a tradition of going out to dinner together after their therapy sessions; at termination, they said that they'd decided to continue the tradition, going out to dinner once a week to spend time together and talk about any relationship issues that had come up during the previous week.

This chapter has presented three approaches to psychotherapy with gay and lesbian couples—approaches that have in common their roots in behavior therapy. These are certainly not the only effective approaches for working with same-sex couples; in fact, recently, there has been an upsurge of literature on same-sex relationships and therapy with same-sex couples (e.g., Clunis & Green, 2000; Green & Mitchell, 2002; Greenan & Tunnell, 2003; Ossana, 2000). The treatment approaches presented in this chapter have the advantage of empirically proven efficacy with heterosexual, married couples; whether their efficacy will be borne out with same-sex couples remains an empirical question worthy of further study.

Chapter 7

Consideration of Other Disorders and Problems

CBT has been applied successfully to many psychological disorders besides depression, anxiety, and relationship distress in couples. Treatment protocols for almost all DSM disorders have been developed from a CBT perspective. In this chapter, we discuss disorders such as posttraumatic stress disorder (PTSD), obsessive–compulsive disorder (OCD), and body dysmorphic disorder, the treatment of which requires similar behavioral and cognitive-behavioral techniques. We discuss psychosocial problems such as substance abuse, and grief and bereavement. Sexual orientation is not the only variable that informs the treatment approach chosen. Therapists need to recognize that cultural background, gender, race, and socioeconomic status all play important roles as well. We provide brief descriptions of the major CBT interventions as applied to the general LGB population.

POSTTRAUMATIC STRESS DISORDER

Lisa had sought CBT after reading a brochure in her physician's office about depression. Over the past 3 months, she had gone through a number of changes and wanted to talk with someone. Her partner, Ingrid, also encouraged Lisa to seek therapy. They had been having difficulty since Lisa had driven across country to visit her family in the Midwest. Since her return from that trip, Lisa was much less sexual and became sullen for no apparent reason. Ingrid had begun to worry about her, and Lisa thought the problems might be a sign of clinical depression.

147

The first two therapy sessions were helpful. Lisa's therapist was skilled at helping her to talk about the symptoms troubling her and to give an account of her history. In the second session, Lisa told her therapist about an incident that occurred when she was 21 years old (she was now 39), which she had believed was long since relegated to the past. She had only recently been reminded of it during her drive to visit her family, through the state of Idaho, where the incident had occurred. When she mentioned the incident in therapy, she began to sob uncontrollably. Her therapist gently said, "I can see this is very hard for you to talk about. It seems like it is quite important, however. Perhaps we can spend an entire session with this on our agenda." Lisa agreed but dreaded the session in which she would need to tell the entire story of what she had, through the years, called "the misjudgment."

By the time Lisa was 21, she had considered herself an "out lesbian" for 1½ years. She had disclosed her sexual orientation to her family and friends in the city in the Midwest where she had been raised, and her family was very supportive. Her parents were well-educated, liberal thinking, schoolteachers. The friends she told during her junior year of college responded that they loved and cared about her. Lisa left the Midwest and moved to a small town in Idaho, because she wanted to take a break prior to applying to graduate school. She liked the mountains and skiing, so she got a job at a ski resort nearby. There were no gay- or lesbian-oriented establishments in the town, but Lisa frequented a local bar, where she felt comfortable with the patrons. One woman in particular, who worked with Lisa at the resort and identified as straight, was very friendly to her at the bar. This woman had a boyfriend who joined them on occasion to have a couple of drinks. One night in early March, the three of them had spent the evening at the bar. Lisa had more to drink than was usually comfortable for her. The man volunteered to drive the two women home. Lisa gave her keys to the woman friend.

The woman lived closest to the bar, so she was dropped off first. Lisa thought that she remembered the man saying, "I'll see you tomorrow morning, honey," but she was uncertain. The man complained of being very tired and a little "high" himself. He said, "You know, my place is just a mile or two away, and you live across town. Why don't you crash on my couch tonight, and we can all have breakfast in the morning." Lisa agreed.

When they arrived at the man's house, which was at the end of a long, deserted drive, he opened the door for her, and they went into his house. She remembered that it was more like a cabin. Lisa did not remember much after that. Soon after they entered the cabin, the man turned on her and punched her hard in the face. She heard him say something about "dykes" and "make a woman out of you." The next thing she recalled was lying face down across a bed with her arms tied to the posts. The man was raping her. He was violent, hurting her. He shouted things like "Are you a woman or a man?"

Lisa did not know how long the ordeal lasted. He had taken out a knife and was holding it to her throat. She recalled having thought that she would die that night. She passed out and awakened the next morning on clean sheets. She was dressed in a clean pair of men's pajamas and had been washed. There was no blood. Her hands were free; she got up to see if the man was still in the cabin. As far as she could tell, she was alone. She found a pair of denim trousers and a sweatshirt folded in a chair by the door, with her car keys and wallet lying on top of them. Her shoes were on the floor. When she took off the pajamas to get into the clothes, she saw that her thighs were bruised, and the pain reminded her of the danger the night before. She could not run because of the discomfort, but walked about 1½ miles down a dirt road before reaching the main highway. She hitched a ride to town to pick up her car, which was parked on the street near the bar, where she had left it the previous night. She was parked across the street from a diner. She saw the man from the night before, with the woman that she thought was her friend, sitting at a table in the diner. They were laughing, and she saw them look directly at her. She got in her car and drove to her apartment. She was too afraid to go to the local police and decided simply to load her things in her car and leave town. She did so, putting a note under her landlady's door, telling her to keep the damage deposit. Lisa drove away from that town and kept driving until she was out of Idaho. Eventually, she sought medical attention but refused to make a police report.

Lisa had never told Ingrid, or any of her family or friends, about the rape. She had tried to put it behind her and not think about it. Within 6 months after the incident, she had applied to graduate school near San Francisco. She thought that she would be safe in a large metropolitan area. She also wanted to live in a city where she would be safe living openly as a lesbian. She met Ingrid in graduate school, and they had fallen in love quickly. They had a commitment ceremony after living together for 2 years. At the time that Lisa started therapy, she and Ingrid had been partners for 15 years.

In this case example, Lisa's therapist at first thought that her problems were primarily due to a major depressive episode. However, it became apparent within the first couple of sessions, while the therapist was completing her case conceptualization, that Lisa was suffering from PTSD. She had successfully kept the memories of the rape at bay for many years, telling no one about the incident. As time went on, she questioned whether she had somehow been partly responsible. She also questioned exactly what had occurred, because she had awakened to find herself in clean pajamas the morning after that terrible night. She had fled the little town in Idaho where the rape occurred and thought that she was leaving behind the memory of the entire incident. However, suppressing her thoughts about the rape came at a terrible price for her.

Like many individuals with PTSD, intrusive thoughts of the traumatic event can be troubling. Lisa had few thoughts during the day, but she was disturbed by nightmares at least once a month. Prior to the rape, Lisa was very outgoing and friendly. Afterward, however, she had become more cautious, particularly around heterosexual students and coworkers. Her fear of the man who had raped her that night generalized to many men, particularly blue-collar workers.

Depending on the setting in which they work, clinicians see a minority of cases reporting the type of trauma Lisa experienced. However, data suggest that young gay men, lesbian women ages 18–24, and LGB college students are victims of violence at rates as high as 22–29% (D'Augelli, 1998). Reports of rape among young lesbian women have been as high as 50% according to the National Lesbian Healthcare Survey (Bradford et al., 1994). Given these statistics and the fact that LGB individuals are often raised in invalidating and hostile environments, clinicians may see LGB clients who present with symptoms of PTSD and either meet full criteria or have certain features of the disorder.

According to DSM-IV (American Psychiatric Association, 1994) PTSD is diagnosed if the person has been exposed to a traumatic event in which he or she "experienced, witnessed, or was confronted with an event or events that involved actual or threatened death or serious injury, or a threat to the physical integrity of self or others" and his or her response involved "intense fear, helplessness or horror" (p. 209). PTSD is diagnosed only if the individual experiences some symptoms of reexperiencing, avoidance, and physiological reactivity. Reexperiencing symptoms can include recurrent and intrusive recollections of the event, distressing dreams, acting or feeling as though the traumatic event were recurring (including dissociation or flashbacks), and intense psychological distress or physiological reactivity when reminded of the event. Avoidance symptoms can include actively trying not to think or talk about the event; avoiding activities, places, or people that remind one of the event; blocking parts of the event out, so that one does not recall an important aspect or aspects of it; losing interest in activities that one enjoyed previously; feeling detached or like an outsider; having a difficult time with strong emotions; feeling numb; and having a sense that one's future may be foreshortened or different.

There also are persistent symptoms of increased arousal that were not present before the traumatic event. This arousal is indicated by problems such as difficulty falling or staying asleep, irritability, angry outbursts, difficulty concentrating, hypervigilance to danger cues, and an exaggerated startle response. Like all DSM disorders, the disturbance must cause clinically significant distress or impaired functioning.

We have presented the diagnostic criteria for PTSD, because the term is frequently overused in clinical parlance (McNally, 2003). Prevalence rates are high, however, with conservative estimates of 20 million people in the United States alone meeting PTSD criteria (Keane, 1998). High incidences of sexual assault on women also make it more likely that therapists working with lesbian or bisexual women will see clients presenting with PTSD. Also, despite discrimination by the Department of Defense, many LGB individuals have served in the military and may have been exposed to combat or other traumatic events during their military duty, resulting in symptoms of PTSD. In our previous example, Lisa met the criteria, because she believed that her life was being threatened, and she was subjected to terrible physical harm. She was terrified during the experience. Lisa moved from the state where the rape occurred, and avoided the cues associated with the rape by residing in a major city as opposed to a rural community. However, she was troubled by feelings of detachment whenever she passed sports bars or playing fields, where groups of men were involved in sports, and she had frequent nightmares. She experienced distress in her sexual relationship with her partner insofar as sex was a cue for traumatic memories. When she was required to return to Idaho, she reexperienced the fear and distress. During sessions with her therapist, Lisa sobbed uncontrollably and experienced brief dissociative periods in which she reported feeling as if she were back in the traumatic situation. During those times, her heart raced, and the palms of her hands felt cold and sweaty.

CBT for PTSD targets the avoidance of the traumatic memories and situational cues. The rationale for treatment is that anxiety reduction, also known as "habituation," has been observed to occur during prolonged exposure (PE) to traumatic memories, and exposure therapy has been shown to be an effective treatment for PTSD in rape victims (Foa, Rothbaum, Riggs, & Murdock, 1991), as well as victims of other traumatic events (Keane, Gerardi, Quinn, & Litz, 1992). Foa, Steketee, and Rothbaum (1989) extended the conceptualization of PTSD, and proposed that PTSD was distinguished from other anxiety disorders because the traumatic event was "of monumental significance, and violated formerly held basic concepts of safety" (p. 166). The development of crime-related PTSD is predicated on the dangerousness of the crime as indicated by perceived threat or extent of physical injury (Kilpatrick et al., 1989).

According to Foa and Kozac (1986), for an exposure to be effective and curative, two things must occur. First, the exposure must invoke the conditioned emotional response—anxiety. Second, through PE, the person must stay in the situation until his or her anxiety goes down—until habituation occurs. This pattern for exposures has actually been proven more effective than exposures in which the stimulus does not cause sufficient anxiety and/or when the client does not habituate because exposure is discontinued too early. If brief exposure to traumatic memories was sufficient, then the intrusive thoughts, nightmares, and so on, experienced as part of the syndrome would serve to reduce anxiety, but this is clearly not the case (Foa et al., 1989). Also, brief exposures to which a client does not habituate can actually reinforce the fear.

Exposure therapy is understandably painful for clients and can be uncomfortable for therapists as well. It is essential to be mindful of the long-term efficacy of the approach in freeing the client from very painful symptoms that would otherwise continue indefinitely. Clients who are reluctant to participate in this treatment can be gently encouraged to tolerate the short-term pain for potential long-term relief. Therapists who are reluctant to undertake this type of therapy can first make sure that they are adequately trained in the approach, and second, realize that this type of therapy may evoke strong emotions in them as well, but that it is all in the service of bringing relief, not further aggravation, to the client.

Exposure sessions usually last from 1½–2 hours (e.g., Foa & Rothbaum, 1998). Multiple sessions during the week are advisable, because prolonged exposure is necessary and also allows the clinician to provide support to the client during a time of increased emotional arousal. The therapist teaches the client to rate the intensity of his or her anxiety, using the Subjective Units of Discomfort Scale[1] (SUDS; Wolpe & Lazarus, 1966, as cited in Nietzel & Bernstein, 1981), which rates the intensity of feared situations from 0 to 100. Exposure begins in session to situations that evoke a moderate level of anxiety, and the client is instructed to stay in the situation until his or her anxiety decreases considerably (i.e., by about 50% of the original SUDS). The exposure sessions are either taped or the client can be asked to write the details of the traumatic situation on paper. Between sessions, homework is assigned, so that clients practice exposure either by listening to the tape or reading the description of the traumatic event. Again, the client should stay in the situation until his or her anxiety has decreased significantly.

Clients are also asked to create an *in vivo* hierarchy of fears, such as going to certain parts of town, being in the presence of men wearing a particular cologne, participating in Fourth of July celebrations, and so on, and the client is asked to expose him- or herself increasingly to such stimuli either with the therapist in session or as homework. In these situations, clients learn to stay in the situation until their anxiety is reduced. This is similar to exposures used in other anxiety disorders, such as social phobia (see Chapter 5), or even simple phobias. Clients with PTSD also frequently avoid many situations that evoke symptoms of PTSD. Lisa, whose story is told at the beginning of this chapter, developed a hierarchy that includes the following:

Situation	SUDS rating
Seeing the man who raped her	100
Being in the town where the rape occurred	90
Getting out of her car anywhere in Idaho	80
Going into small-town bars or pubs	70
Stopping at rural convenience stores	60
Being surrounded by men at a sporting event	50
Walking down a dirt road in daytime	40
Walking with friends down a dark city street	30
Going on a day hike in a rural area	20
Driving on rural highways	10

The benefits of exposure treatment are apparent in cases involving other kinds of trauma as well. For example, David suffered from PTSD symptoms after seeing several of his friends die in the hospital from complications due to AIDS, following his own traumatic experience and subsequent medical treatment of a painful, severe, leg burn that occurred on his job. He was able to return to work but avoided hospitals and refused to even watch television shows depicting medical procedures. His avoidance became problematic, because he had not received a medical checkup in 5 years. His therapist began *in vivo* exposure exercises by taking David on excursions to a nearby hospital, first going to the gift shop, to the cafeteria, and then through the wards. David was also instructed to watch movies in which doctors and hospitals were featured prominently in the plot. Content of imaginal exposure exercises for David included, first, watching his closest friend, Ed, during the last days of Ed's life in an intensive care unit, and second, imagining his own treatment for his burns.

As discussed earlier, PE can be very evocative for both therapist and client. Therefore, we strongly recommend that clinicians seek training in the techniques by attending workshops and professional presentations. Furthermore, clinicians, supervised by an expert, should treat one or two clients for PTSD prior to conducting PE solo. Experts in the area of PTSD have also advocated utilization of multidimensional treatment, including both cognitive and behavioral components (e.g., Resick & Schnicke, 1992). PE is a major component of these treatments, but they also include techniques for teaching clients to manage anxiety and cognitive restructuring components. Cognitive restructuring focuses on the client's assessment of danger in situations that were neutral prior to the traumatic event. Resick and Schnicke suggest that pretrauma beliefs about safety may give way to posttrauma beliefs about the world as a more dangerous place or a decrease in belief in one's competence. These beliefs must also be addressed in therapy.

Clinicians with little PE experience may worry that a treatment requiring clients to reexperience their trauma through imaginal exposure may exacerbate symptoms of PTSD. Foa, Zoellner, Feeny, Hembree, and Alvarez-Conrad (2002) addressed this concern in an analysis of PE treatment for female rape victims. Using measures of PTSD, depression, and anxiety throughout a course of treatment with PE, they found that the majority of participants did not have an exacerbation of PTSD or depression after the initiation of PE. For the minority of participants who experienced a temporary exacerbation of PTSD or depressive symptoms, the increase in symptoms did follow initiation of PE. Foa et al. found a statistically significant relationship between initiation of PE and an increase in anxiety symptoms. However, exacerbation of symptoms was not related to treatment outcome, and those who experienced an exacerbation of symptoms did not benefit less from treatment than those who did not show such exacerbation. Nor did the individuals who dropped out of treatment experience exacerbation of symptoms at higher rates than treatment completers. The authors concluded that for female rape survivors treated with PE for PTSD, initiation of PE did not increase negative symptoms. They cautioned, however, that their results might not generalize to other groups of PTSD patients.

PE remains the most well-documented behavioral treatment for PTSD. Recently, however, Resick, Nishith, Weaver, Astin, and Feuer (2002) compared cognitive processing therapy (CPT) with PE and found that CPT is as effective in the treatment of female rape survivors suffering from PTSD. PE is a component of the CPT treatment package, but clients are only required to write about their rape and discuss the details of the rape twice during the course of therapy, as opposed to PE, in which imaginal exposure is repeated over the course of treatment.

This therefore may increase many clients' willingness to participate in the treatment. Resick and colleagues found that CPT is as effective as PE in treatment of PTSD, and that both treatments are superior to a minimal attention control. CPT, however, is superior to PE in the treatment of trauma-related guilt. Participants in the Resick et al. study varied relative to duration of PTSD symptoms, and many had comorbid personality disorders or other psychiatric diagnoses. Given the diversity of their sample, the authors concluded that their results would likely generalize to types of trauma other than rape, and to a broader group of clients than female rape survivors.

OBSESSIVE–COMPULSIVE DISORDER

OCD is characterized by obsessive fears or intrusive thoughts (e.g., of contamination, death, being responsible for injury of others) and the ritualized compulsive behaviors that reduce the fear. Obsessions are unwanted, intrusive thoughts or images that evoke anxiety, and compulsions are voluntary thoughts (e.g., counting, praying) or behaviors (e.g., repeatedly checking, seeking reassurance) that neutralize the anxiety (Salkovskis & Kirk, 1996). Although these thoughts cause significant distress, usually clients recognize that the content of the compulsion is unreasonable, unrealistic, or even absurd (if not, there is a diagnostic specifier, "with poor insight," and CBT is much more difficult to do) Most people think of compulsive hand washers when they think of OCD. Many OCD clients do have contamination fears, but a variety of fears and obsessions not connected to contamination can also lead to the diagnosis.

In general, the cognitive-behavioral treatment of OCD shares elements with CBT for other anxiety disorders and PTSD. The treatment, therefore, consists of exposure to the objects of fear, either *in vivo* or through imagery, while preventing the ritualistic behaviors, hence the name "exposure with response prevention" (ERP) therapy (see Abramowitz & Kalsy, 2001, for a review of current treatments). Just as with other disorders, fear hierarchies must be developed with the use of a SUDS scale. ERP begins with an item of moderate intensity on the SUDS scale. Cognitive components such as faulty premises, underlying beliefs, and erroneous rules of inference may hinder information processing and prevent alleviation of the fear (Foa & Kozak, 1986).

Therapists are occasionally confronted with people who identify as heterosexual but maintain obsessive fears that that they are gay (e.g., Phillipson, 2002). Typically, the individual with this type of obsession is a young adult male. In many cases, the individual has gay or lesbian friends and does not show signs of homophobia or morbid fears of LGB people. Still others are afraid of the implications of being gay and may never have met a gay person. There is a difference between a man who looks at other men with sexual interest and/or sexual arousal and one who looks at other men and wonders if he's gay. Men with this particular form of OCD worry that they are gay, or may become gay, simply by thinking about it a lot. They mistake their checking to see whether they are attracted to men or have sexual feelings as a sign that they are gay. Often, these types of men can point to no particular sign of attraction, although they spend a lot of time worrying about the possibility of becoming gay. Often, their only behavior that is suggestive of being gay is their gaze toward men to see whether they are attracted. It is therefore a checking function rather than an appetitive one. These men are different from a man who may in fact be questioning his sexual orientation and clearly feels aroused. Kuehlwein (personal communication, May 4, 2002) suggests that therapists should provide information for clients in this situation about what sorts of things we, as professionals, would expect if the person were gay or bisexual and, alternatively, what we'd expect if he (or in rarer cases, she) were straight but suffering from OCD. Making two columns and then comparing these to the actual situation can help the client to see which of the two is more likely. If the individual were LGB and uncertain, for example, we'd expect significant physical attraction to members of the same sex, and that his or her sexual dreams would frequently include members of the same sex. Fantasies would also frequently include members of the same sex. If the person were suffering from OCD, we'd expect he or she would frequently worry about being aroused but experience little actual arousal. When the content of obsessions is about sexual orientation, male clients often report being concerned about imagining another man's penis, looking at someone in the shower at a gymnasium or public pool, or having a dream with male sexual content. As with other OCD clients, there is thought–act fusion: the belief that thoughts somehow equate to actions, that thinking = doing. Therefore, their preoccupation with the gay possibility is itself a sign that they may be gay. The more they worry about this dreaded result, the more they feel the need to check, thereby making the concept loom larger in their minds.

Some clients present with pure obsessions, without the component ritualized or compulsive behaviors. However, frequently, clients who appear to be obsessive, without compulsive behaviors, engage in covert (i.e., mental) neutralizing behaviors (Salkovskis & Kirk, 1996) that must be attended to in treatment. For example, Dillon worried that he might be gay. He spent up to 5 hours a day ruminating over thoughts such as "What if I'm gay. I noticed the bulge in that guy's pants. I must be gay." Dillon had two very dear friends who were gay men, and he spent a great deal of time with them. He did not try to avoid looking at them, nor did he engage in other overt behaviors to neutralize his fears. However, when he had the thought, "I saw the bulge in that guy's pants," he would immediately imagine women's breasts and try to neutralize the "gay" thought with thoughts about women's bodies. Dillon, like many OCD sufferers, engaged in neutralizing behaviors in the form of thinking. Clinicians need to ask questions skillfully to assess whether clients have covert responses to neutralize their anxiety about their obsessions. It would have been easy to think that Dillon was obsessive without compulsive behavior, but this would not be true. He did not engage in overt behaviors but did, indeed, engage in covert ones.

Salkovskis and Kirk (1996) recommend two treatment components for treating obsessions without covert compulsive behaviors. First, the client must be repeatedly exposed to the obsessive thought. This can be accomplished by having the client write the thought repeatedly, or taping the thought on a loop tape. For Dillon, the thought, "I might be gay. There is a chance that I could be gay," was the evocative thought. Repeating this thought to himself created a great deal of distress for Dillon. He rated his SUDS at 75 when first composing the dialogue. Dillon was assigned practice at home, to listen to the tape for at least 1 hour, twice daily. He was to listen until his anxiety decreased by at least 50%. He reported that his anxiety only decreased by 10% on the first three trials of the homework. However, he persisted in doing the exposure, and by the end of the week, his anxiety was reduced to SUDS of 20 on three trials. Salkovskis and Kirk recommend that generalization be programmed into the treatment by instructing the client to listen to the tape in a difficult situation and also while anxious, and by varying the taped habituation either by using a nonlooped tape, varying the thought contents, or even by introducing loud noises into the tape to induce startle responses (p. 162). Notice that the client is asked to repeat the thought without engaging in the neutralizing covert behaviors (in this case, thinking about women's bodies).

BODY DYSMORPHIC DISORDER

Gay culture is filled with images of youth and beauty. Films, magazine covers, and advertisements developed for gay male audiences contain images of young, muscled, slender men (just as material aimed at heterosexual men contains similar images of young women). There is limited empirical evidence (Siever, 1994), and much clinical and anecdotal evidence to suggest that gay men suffer from eating disorders at rates similar to those of heterosexual women, who also face pressure to be thin, young, and beautiful. Body dysmorphic disorder, defined as a morbid concern with perceived inperfections in one's appearance, is often associated with eating disorders. Siever found that gay men and heterosexual women suffer from higher incidence of eating disorders than either lesbians or heterosexual men. Although, in this chapter, we emphasize the issue as it pertains to gay men, clearly, lesbians, as women, are not immune to the pressures of society to remain youthful and beautiful (Cogan, 1999). Although feminist perspectives on health and beauty have discouraged adherence to male-dominated standards, the media and the dominant culture still confront lesbians and bisexual women with unrealistic images of femininity and youth. Bisexual women feel more pressure regarding their appearance when their partner is male (Taub, 1999).

In the case of body dysmorphic disorder, the target of treatment is obsessive concern with physical flaws in the absence of objective data that any real physical deformity outside of normal limits exists. Compulsive behaviors that may accompany body dysmorphic disorder include checking the area of dissatisfaction (e.g., looking in mirrors, touching parts of the body, seeking feedback from others); excessive exercise or food restriction; using drugs, such as anabolic steroids, to change body type; or having plastic surgery to fix perceived physical defects. An individual would not receive a diagnosis of body dysmorphic disorder if he or she were concerned about a physical abnormality judged by common standards to indeed deviate from the norm, such as someone concerned about a disfiguring scar from an accident.

Rosen (1995) suggested that CBT for body dysmorphic disorder should consist of both cognitive restructuring and behavioral procedures. The client is asked to self-monitor using thought records in situations in which body image is of concern, and to record the thoughts and beliefs associated with such situations. For example, Alicia was concerned that she was losing her hair. Although her hair was thin, hair loss was not noticeable. She believed that a woman without thick hair was unattractive. Alicia also believed that she would be completely bald in a short time and would need to wear wigs. She recognized that some women in her community actually shaved their heads, or had tattoos on their scalp. She considered this very unattractive, however, and equated such a look with underemployment and sexual aggressiveness. Her self-monitoring records suggested that she was vulnerable to distress in situations in which she saw another woman or man with thick hair and compared herself to them. She would think, "They look wonderful, and you can see my scalp through my hair." Alicia tried to cope with her anxiety by engaging in behaviors that temporarily reduced it but, ultimately, maintained her concern with her hair. She would then look for people with thinner hair, usually elderly women, and if she were with friends, she'd ask them if her hair was "as thin as that." She also counted the hairs that fell in her sink or shower.

Eddie, a 30-year-old, gay white man, had more global bodily concerns. He believed that he would only meet another man and find a partner if he were buff like the models he saw in magazines. He had been overweight as a young boy, and his father called him "Chubbo." When Eddie saw himself in the mirror, he saw a flabby, out-of-shape man. In truth, he was very fit, and was mistaking muscle tone for fat. Ironically, Eddie's belief was reinforced by the fact that he was frequently asked out by men he met at the gym. He would talk with these men in the locker room after a workout, and because they asked him out after he had completed a vigorous workout, he believed that they were only interested in him because he was "pumped." This was also the case when he went out to clubs. He would only go out if he had spent at least 2 hours at the gym that day. Like Alicia, Eddie also looked at men he thought were overweight and would ask friends, "Does my body look like that?" He worked out 7 days a week, for at least 2 hours, if not more. Therapy for Eddie consisted of monitoring his thoughts and also of dealing with the behavioral manifestations of the disorder.

Some clients have difficulty identifying automatic thoughts as they arise. If this is the case, Rosen (1995) suggests that therapists provide clients with questionnaires that help them to identify situations in which they are uncomfortable, and their self-criticism. He suggests the Body Image Automatic Thoughts Questionnaire (Cash, 1991, as cited in Rosen, 1995) or the Situational Inventory of Body-Image Dysphoria (Cash, 1994, as cited in Rosen, 1995). Therapists can also assist clients in the session to identify automatic thoughts that occur while in the presence of the therapist.

Rosen (1995) suggests that therapists should not get into arguments with clients regarding their beliefs and attitudes. He points out that some degree of dissatisfaction with one's body is normal, and that the maladaptive thoughts of clients with body dysmorphic disorder are not likely to be completely extinguished. In Alicia's case, for example, her therapist would say, "Well, yes, your hair is not as thick as some peoples," but she would help Alicia to find alternatives to the catastrophic conclusions that she drew regarding this. Instead of thinking, "I'll be completely bald," Alicia would counter her automatic thought by telling herself, "Like many women, my hair may get thinner with age, but it is not likely to completely fall out."

Behaviorally, the therapist can help clients expose themselves to the situations that cause anxiety, without engaging in the behaviors that temporarily reduce the anxiety. To facilitate adherence to the treatment, therapists typically do this in a stepwise manner, by starting with exposure to stimuli that elicit only a moderate amount of distress. For example, Alicia was asked to walk past people with thin hair and not ask her friends if she looked like them. Eddie was instructed to spend time looking at himself in the mirror in the morning but to refrain from pinching and squeezing the flesh in his midsection to "assess whether he was getting fatter." He was not, however, asked to go out to a club without having gone to the gym, or to lessen his workout times. The latter would have caused a great deal of distress and needed to be kept as an exposure exercise later in therapy.

In the cases of both Alicia and Eddie, neither was completely free of concerns about appearance. However, therapy helped them to discontinue some of the dysfunctional thinking and behavior that exacerbated their concerns. After therapy was completed, Alicia continued to have concerns about her hair, but she had reduced her obsessive rumination significantly and was spending 50% less time fixing her hair to cover up perceived inadequacies. Likewise, Eddie was not completely cured. He was still concerned about looking good and maintained a fear of getting fat. Therapy, however, helped to prevent further harm by allowing Eddie to decide that he would not consider using steroids. He also reduced his activity at the gym to five times per week, and limited his workout time to 1–1½ hours. This allowed him to spend more time with friends and pursue avocational goals that he had been unable to prior to therapy because of time constraints.

PHYSICAL ILLNESS AND BEREAVEMENT

A close friend of one of the authors (Martell), who was living with, and ultimately dying from, complications due to AIDS, would quote the title from Jim Morrison's biography *Nobody Gets Out of Here Alive* to point out humorously that death and dying are inevitable. Human beings are vulnerable to a variety of illnesses and injuries, and death is a part of life for us all. In the gay male community, HIV/AIDS has taken on special significance, although it is not the only physical problem faced by gay men. In the United States and Europe, disproportionate numbers of gay and bisexual men have been affected by HIV/AIDS, and the LGB community mobilized around this health threat from the early 1980s, when government resources were scarce. Lesbians, however, are at no greater risk for any particular health problem than are heterosexual or bisexual women. In fact, they are at less risk of cervical cancer than heterosexual or bisexual women, who have a greater chance of being exposed to sexually transmitted diseases, although they may be at greater risk of breast cancer if they delay childbirth, never become pregnant, or bear and breast-feed children (Kauth, Hartwig, & Kalichman, 2000).

For the individual living with an illness, there are several points at which help from behavioral health providers may be sought: (1) soon after initial diagnosis, (2) during a time of increased symptomatology, (3) during remission of symptoms and resumption of normal life routines, or (4) near the end of life. Families and loved ones may seek help at these times as well, as well as after the death of a significant other. During some of these stages, clients may require support and empathy more than any other intervention. Yet cognitive-behavioral interventions are particularly helpful for problems that can arise during any of these stages. In this section, we present several short vignettes that demonstrate the unique concerns of LGB people facing these challenging life problems, and the CBT interventions that can be useful in helping them. Because medical research continues to uncover new treatments and controversies in the treatment of HIV and of breast cancer, clinicians must be aware that the concerns of clients in the 2000s may not be the same as those of clients later in the century. This has certainly been the case with HIV/AIDS. In 1985, people with a diagnosis of AIDS had a prognosis of approximately 2 years prior to death. Since 1995, after the discovery of the protease inhibitors, people able to tolerate these powerful drugs are living with AIDS for many years, and the disease is being treated as a chronic, life-threatening condition rather than a terminal illness.

Researchers since the early 1990s have found that active coping strategies are related to better adjustment following a diagnosis of HIV/AIDS (e.g., Pakenham, Dadds, & Terry, 1994). Coping strategies such as optimism, control, and action, and interpersonal coping strategies have been shown to be related to low levels of global and illness-related distress (Pakenham et al., 1994). Teaching such coping strategies has been the realm of CBT since its inception. Keeping in mind that several factors affect response to illness, including type of illness, availability of social support, cultural background, age, and individual history, we now turn to a discussion of several cognitive-behavioral interventions at each of the stages of illness.

After Initial Diagnosis

The time following an initial diagnosis of a medical illness is particularly crucial. A person diagnosed with a chronic or life-threatening illness must make a variety of cognitive shifts to cope with this life challenge. Such a diagnosis shakes the individual's sense of well-being, and many people begin to see differences in themselves and the world prior to and following diagnosis. After a diagnosis, the world may be perceived as dangerous or threatening. The person may define him- or herself as a patient or as damaged in some way. The necessity of medical treatment reinforces the idea of the person as a "patient" and can engender feelings of dependence and vulnerability. Ideas about being damaged may be particularly salient in individuals dealing with illnesses, such as HIV, that have negative societal stigma (Herek, 1999), or, in the case of breast cancer, that may require treatment that is difficult or disfiguring.

As part of a thorough assessment, therapists should assess the client's perception of the medical community. Lesbian clients, for example, may see the medical community as patriarchal and may neglect regular medical care (Kauth et al., 2000). It is important to appreciate that many LGB clients may also have experienced prejudice in the medical system, so their concerns may be founded in reality. Many gay male or bisexual male clients' fear of talking to heterosexual doctors about same-sex sexual practices can allow medical problems to remain undiagnosed. Although intermittent periods of denial can be helpful in coping with a chronic illness (Taylor & Aspinwall, 1990), clients who use denial as a primary coping strategy may neglect necessary medical attention and place themselves at greater risk for complications. Insofar as fear and distrust of the medical establishment lead to denial and avoidance, clients can fail to seek out and receive the medical care necessary to survive a life-threatening illness. Clients seeking therapy after an initial diagnosis of a major illness may benefit from cognitive restructuring to counter hopelessness about the diagnosis or fears of the medical system. Therapists must keep in mind the reality of the prejudice against LGB individuals that exists in the medical establishment, however, and need to maintain empathic objectivity in helping clients develop a balanced understanding of their situation postdiagnosis.

Enrique, a 22-year-old, Latino gay man tested seropositive for HIV 1 week prior to seeking therapy. He was comfortable with his doctor, who was an openly gay family practice physician, and had sufficient health insurance to pay for necessary treatments. Enrique had become very depressed, however, on hearing the news that he was HIV-positive, and his physician had referred him for therapy. Enrique's greatest fear, understandably, was that his life would be foreshortened and he would suffer a painful death. In discussions with his physician, he had decided not to take any medications, because his blood work looked good, with the exception of being HIV-seropositive. In the following exchange, Enrique's therapist uses cognitive restructuring to help him to understand his illness more broadly, and not as the death sentence he believed it to be.

THERAPIST: There are many concerns that someone would have after hearing the news you have just received. Could you tell me some of your thoughts over the past week?

ENRIQUE: Mostly, I just think, "I'm going to die," and although I've always known everybody is going to die, I didn't ever think about it before now.

THERAPIST: Well, at age 22, death is not usually what one thinks about. How soon do you fear you will die?

ENRIQUE: Well, I know people live longer now with HIV than in the past, and my doctor tells me that I am healthy otherwise. I don't know, I just feel like I could drop dead at any time.

THERAPIST: Do you know anyone who has died as a result of AIDS?

ENRIQUE: No, I only know a few guys who are HIV-positive.

THERAPIST: Are you very close to these guys?

ENRIQUE: One of them is a very good friend. We hang out a lot. He is a little older than me—he's 31.

THERAPIST: Do you know how long he has known he is HIV-positive?

ENRIQUE: I think he told me he's known since about 1993.

THERAPIST: So that would have made him about your age when he first found out, correct?

ENRIQUE: Yeah, I guess so.

THERAPIST: Do you know how his health is?

ENRIQUE: Well, he is taking medication that makes him a little sick, but he is generally healthy. He and I go hiking a lot and dancing; he's able to do both without trouble.

THERAPIST: Do you think of him as someone who is dying?

ENRIQUE: No, I see him as someone who is living with an illness, and one that doesn't seem to affect him too much, so far as I can tell.

THERAPIST: Have you ever spoken to him about how his illness affects him?

ENRIQUE: No.

THERAPIST: Well, it may affect him in ways that he doesn't discuss, but I think it is important that you don't see him as someone who is dying. But that has been your primary thought about yourself over the past week.

ENRIQUE: Well, it is what really scares me.

THERAPIST: Yes, I understand that. I think dying scares all of us. Being afraid after hearing that you are HIV-positive is normal and understandable. However, when you think, "I'm going to die," you are kind of predicting the future, aren't you?

ENRIQUE: Yes, but it seems like a realistic prediction.

THERAPIST: It is a realistic prediction for everyone, because that is the ultimate outcome of life for us all. I know what you mean, though, that for you it seems more immediate.

ENRIQUE: Yes. I feel like I've really blown it, and now I'm not going to grow old.

THERAPIST: Have you ever heard of people who are growing old with HIV?

ENRIQUE: Well, I know Magic Johnson has had HIV for a long time, and he's still alive.

THERAPIST: Yes, and I can tell you that I've worked with a great deal of men who are HIV-positive, and many of them have been living with HIV for 20 years or more.

ENRIQUE: Well, that would make me 42 when it finally gets me.

THERAPIST: Well, here we are in 2002, and people are living with HIV or AIDS for decades. Do you know how long people lived with AIDS back in 1992?

ENRIQUE: No.

THERAPIST: I would say that the average was 2 or 3 years. So a lot has changed in the past 10 years, hasn't it?

ENRIQUE: I guess so.

THERAPIST: So if so much has changed in 10 years, do you think that there will continue to be medical advances over the next few decades?

ENRIQUE: I hope so.

THERAPIST: What do you think is likely to happen?

ENRIQUE: Well, even if there isn't a cure, they will find better medicines.

THERAPIST: Yes, that is what has been happening, so do you think that will continue?

ENRIQUE: I think so.

THERAPIST: If that continues, what is the likely outcome for you?

ENRIQUE: I'll be on medicines, but I'll live a long time.

THERAPIST: How much do you believe that?

ENRIQUE: I guess I'm 50/50.

THERAPIST: Were you 50/50 about the belief that you were going to die over the past week?

ENRIQUE: No, I think I was convinced I was dying.

THERAPIST: How do you feel now, being 50/50?

ENRIQUE: Scared, still really scared. I think I'm more hopeful, though.

THERAPIST: So why don't we spend a little time today talking about how you can help yourself to feel more hopeful when you start to think that you are going to die? Do you think that would be helpful for you right now?

ENRIQUE: Yes, I guess so.

In this example, the therapist does not take an overly optimistic attitude about life and death. However, the therapist works with the client to counteract the pessimistic attitude contributing to Enrique's depressive reaction to the news that he was HIV-positive. Also, the therapist works from the premise that being scared and distressed about learning that one is HIV-positive is normal. The therapist gently questions Enrique's absolute belief that he is going to die, and helps him to see that there are people living with rather than dying from HIV. The therapist will later teach Enrique to use cognitive restructuring, perhaps with the help of thought records, to develop coping responses to his frightening thoughts.

Martha was different from Enrique. She was 49 years old, Caucasian, and had been in a committed relationship with a woman for the past 20 years. Her partner was a nutritionist. Martha owned and operated a small lawn and garden shop. She believed in alternative medicine and had given birth to her only daughter naturally, with the help of a midwife at a birthing center, and she received medical treatment from a naturopathic physician. When she found a lump in her right breast, her naturopath referred her to a female gynecologist for physical examination. The gynecologist had referred her to a male oncologist. Martha was distressed by the likely diagnosis of breast cancer but also fearful of becoming a pawn of a male-dominated medical system. She responded to this in her therapy session:

MARTHA: I can't believe this is happening to me. I've taken such good care of myself, and I've always been in control of my health care. Now I'm going to be another statistic in the ranks of countless women who have been pushed around by the system. I'm mad at Joan [her naturopathic doctor] for giving me so little advice about what to expect regarding treatments.

THERAPIST: It sounds to me like you expect the worst when it comes to treatment.

MARTHA: Well, what do men know about this anyway? They can cut out lumps or cut off breasts, but they don't have to experience any of it!

THERAPIST: So you are concerned that the oncologist you've been referred to is a man?

MARTHA: I'm concerned that he's a man and that he's an oncologist.

THERAPIST: Would you rather see a woman?

MARTHA: She'd still be an oncologist and have the same training. I think I'd be more comfortable in terms of the actual procedures, but she'd still be part of the system.

THERAPIST: Did you ask for a referral to a woman?

MARTHA: Yes, but this guy is considered the best by my gynecologist, and several acquaintances also know about him and say he has an excellent reputation.

THERAPIST: Do you feel confident about his reputation?

MARTHA: Yes, but not his profession.

THERAPIST: So you have lots of concerns about the medical profession. Would it be helpful if you and I talked about some of your specific concerns regarding your care?

MARTHA: I'm not sure what you mean.

THERAPIST: Well, it sounds like you are going to go and see this oncologist. You also are worried about being victimized by the system. Perhaps we could consider some of your concerns and discuss ways that you can have some control over what happens to you.

MARTHA: I see. Well, my first concern is that they are going to want to do surgery right away.

THERAPIST: Will you ask them what the alternatives are?

MARTHA: I suppose I could, but even though I seem tough, when I get into the doctors' office, and they give me bad news, my head swims and I just say "yes" to whatever they suggest.

THERAPIST: Would you like to write down some questions you could ask the doctor?

MARTHA: That might help.

THERAPIST: So let's start with "What alternatives do I have to surgery?" Can you think of other concerns?

MARTHA: I really want to try to deal with this in ways that I've dealt with other health issues. I'm afraid that the doctor will just tell me to do what he says and forget alternative treatments.

THERAPIST: What alternative treatments are you thinking about?

MARTHA: Maybe taking a naturopathic remedy of some sort.

THERAPIST: So would you like to ask the doctor if there would be any contraindications in taking such remedies? This way, you will let him know that you intend to continue to see your naturopath, but that you also are considering possible complications.

MARTHA: That would be good.

In this exchange, note that the therapist is not challenging Martha's belief regarding the medical establishment at this point. Instead, she talks Martha through steps that might give her a better sense of control of her care. Once Martha has seen the oncologist, there may be an opportunity for cognitive restructuring to weigh the evidence that supports or does not support her belief that he will be patriarchal, unresponsive to her needs, and indifferent to her distress.

Another issue that people face upon receiving a medical diagnosis, particularly of illnesses that carry with them certain social stigmas, such as AIDS or cancer, is when and whom to tell. For gay and bisexual men, this becomes a particularly salient concern when they discover that they are HIV-positive. Many anti-gay groups hold men who have sex with men responsible for the AIDS epidemic (Herek & Capitanio, 1999). Frequently, these men hesitate telling family and friends about their diagnosis for fear of blame being cast on them. In some cases, the HIV diagnosis is an impetus for a client to come out to his family of origin, although he may choose not to disclose his seropositive status. People with chronic illnesses usually do not want to worry their families. CBT therapists can help people in making decisions about who and when to tell by developing specific lists of pros and cons of telling particular individuals. Such lists should include, as much as the client knows, the person's reactions to being told similar news in the past, or to the client in general. The client's ability to cope with the response of the other person should also be considered when developing a list of pros and cons.

Therapists who work with clients living with chronic or life-threatening illnesses can be helpful partners in care. CBT therapists can help clients to develop routines that help them to remain compliant with medication, as well as to learn coping strategies, such as relaxation training, to help mitigate some of the physical distress caused by a number of medications. It is important that people living with a chronic illness continue to remain hopeful and to engage in health-promoting behaviors. Therefore, the CBT therapist can also assist clients in learning about and maintaining proper nutrition and exercise, and refraining from excessive use of alcohol and nonprescription drugs. During periods of exacerbation of symptoms, the therapist can take a particularly active role in the client's care.

Periods of Exacerbated Medical Symptoms

When clients face an increase in physical symptoms or deterioration in health, CBT therapists can assist them in several ways. First, helping the clients to balance fears and worries with alternative coping statements can allow them to maintain an attitude of calm in the midst of great challenges. Second, therapists can help clients to set priorities in their lives, such as making decisions about balancing work and time with loved ones, or going out on disability leave. Again, evaluating pros and cons of decisions is a basic, and helpful tool. Third, when clients feel physically worse, they may become passive and fail to express preferences and concerns to medical personnel. The CBT therapist can help clients to practice assertiveness and ask for what they wish, when dealing with the medical community. Therapists can also use cognitive restructuring to counter the client's hopelessness and beliefs that he or she is helpless to control his or her own medical care (Gluhoski, 1996). Fourth, the CBT therapist can help clients problem-solve about seeking assistance from loved ones, and from the community at large. Finally, the therapist can teach self-soothing skills and help clients to develop self-care behaviors to assist them to cope in times of increased physical distress.

Periods of Remission and Resumption of Normal Life Routines

Thankfully, diseases do go into remission. Such is frequently the case with cancers that respond to treatment. In the case of HIV, although the disease itself does not remit, clients can respond quite well to treatment and maintain undetectable levels of the virus over long periods of time. Therapists may be called on during these times to help clients reshape their view of themselves. Now, rather than being "patients," they must recognize themselves as survivors. This requires another cognitive shift. Anxiety and worry about a foreshortened life may remain, however, even in the case of remission of illness. Clients may become well enough to return to the workforce after long periods of disability. Fears of failure, stigmatization, or incompetence can be addressed with cognitive restructuring, behavioral experiments, and guided activity. Clients can learn to take steps toward ultimate goals rather than trying to jump back into life, as if they had never been sick. People who remain ill, but whose symptoms have remitted to the point that they can return to some form of gainful work, may first begin with volunteer opportunities, so that they don't jeopardize disability benefits that may be needed should they suffer a recurrence of symptoms.

Near the End of Life

CBT therapists who do not work in medical settings are less likely to deal with clients in the end stages of terminal illness. During this time of life, people usually turn to family or clergy for solace, and are often in the hands of the medical community. LGB persons facing the end of life may not turn to traditional sources. Family may not be supportive, and it is important that LGB individuals clearly indicate through living wills and powers of attorney whom they will allow to make medical decisions should they be incapacitated. Therapists should encourage clients to seek legal advice long before it is necessary for someone to make decisions about end-of-life care. Many LGB people have left organized religious groups because of the discriminatory attitudes and behaviors toward homosexuality and bisexuality that continue in most religions. Fears about the afterlife, spiritual interests, or concerns about the meaning of life do not subside, however, just because someone does not attend religious services. For a majority of people who will have such concerns, the end of life is a time that will elicit them. Secular therapists may therefore sometimes be asked to take the role traditionally held by clergy and chaplains. Sitting at the bedsides of dying persons, the CBT therapist can review their lives with them: what makes them feel proud, what they wish had been different. He or she can also look for small ways to increase their comfort or allay fears. For example, in one situation, a CBT therapist was called in to help a young man with AIDS, who was very anxious in the last days of his life. He had no family and refused to see clergy in the hospital. His physician did not believe that increasing antianxiety medications was indicated. The therapist asked the client what he feared most. The young man was not afraid of dying, because he thought he would see his beloved grandmother. However, he did not want to leave his life behind. The therapist asked him to tell about his life and tried to help him to shift the focus from his fear of losing his life to his appreciation of the life he had lived, with all the positive and negative aspects discussed in as much detail as the client could manage in his weakened state. Also, the young man worried that he wasn't getting oxygen. The therapist removed the nasal canula from the client's nose, so that the airflow could be felt on the client's upper lip, pointing out to him that he could try to feel the air blowing out of the tubes or listen to the sound of the air in the tubes to reassure himself that he was getting proper oxygen. The therapist also asked the nurses to remind the client that he could rely on the machines to work for him. Staying at the bedside of a dying patient is not usually where therapists find themselves. However, being open to doing so for an LGB client who does not have other resources is a rewarding opportunity for therapists working with these individuals.

SUBSTANCE ABUSE TREATMENT

CBT offers a view of substance abuse treatment that runs counter to the popular 12-step models. Although many individuals who do have drug or alcohol abuse problems appear to benefit from abstinence and 12-step programs, others do not, and CBT offers help for those individuals.

There is a common belief that there is a higher incidence of substance use, although not of substance dependence, in LGB communities. This population may be more likely to accept experimentation with various drugs as socially appropriate than heterosexual counterparts. However, after a review of the literature, Bux (1996) concluded that there was little evidence to support the belief that lesbians and gay men are more likely to be problem drinkers than are heterosexual men and women. A review of the literature on substance use and abuse rates in the LGB community is beyond the scope of this chapter. However, suffice it to say that early surveys, conducted from samples of lesbians or gay men recruited in bars, overstated the problem of substance abuse in the LGB community (Bux, 1996). Nevertheless some LGB individuals do have substance abuse problems. Furthermore, substance abuse among gay men and bisexual men and women is of particular concern because of increased risk of HIV infection and, for those already infected, detrimental effects on health status. People under the influence can also make very bad decisions in a variety of contexts (such as meeting someone for sex in a dangerous place). A harm reduction model (Marlatt, Larimer, Baer, & Quigley, 1993) is particularly useful in this regard.

Harm reduction is based on the assumption that habits fall along a continuum of harmful consequences (Roberts & Marlatt, 1999) and that steps can be taken to intervene in the environment and with the individual to reduce the risk of harmful consequences. Harm reduction is not antiabstinence; therefore, it is not contrary to 12-step models. It recognizes abstinence as an ideal but offers an alternative for those who will not or cannot currently abstain to reduce harm from their substance use (Roberts & Marlatt, 1999). Therapists working from a harm reduction model use the nonconfrontational method of motivational interviewing (Miller & Rollnick, 2002) to assist clients to come to their own decisions about the need to change their behavior. Harm reduction techniques vary broadly but include programs such as providing condoms in community clinics and needle-exchange programs. The goal in harm reduction is to treat clients as individuals capable of making their own decisions, given proper information relevant to their particular situation, and to help them to recognize behaviors that they may consider problematic. They are then taught how to reduce harmful behaviors. Programs of relapse prevention (Marlatt, 1985) can help individuals to cope with high-risk situations. Roberts and Marlatt (1998) recommend the following guidelines for relapse prevention:

1. Reframe relapse as a process in which setbacks can be viewed as opportunities for learning rather than as failure situations.
2. Identify high-risk situations that include environmental occurrence, interpersonal interactions, or internal factors such as affect, cognitions, or physiological states.
3. Teach clients how to cope with urges by using coping behaviors such as "urge surfing" and reminding themselves of potentially negative consequences.
4. Teach clients to learn from experience to minimize the negative consequences of relapse.
5. Help clients achieve lifestyle balance by replacing addictive behaviors with other sources of pleasurable activity and maintaining moderation.

Harm reduction and relapse prevention may be particularly useful to LGB individuals for several reasons. First, for a group already suffering from stigmatization and prejudice, a harm reduction model removes the stigma of illness and disease from substance abuse, conceptualizing it as a problem rather than a habit. Second, many LGB individuals who reject 12-step programs do so on the basis of the religious overtones of such programs. Harm reduction and relapse prevention models do not propose that clients rely on a "higher power," but instead teach self-control skills to the individuals. They respect the ability of individuals to make informed decisions rather than insisting that they *should* take any particular course of behavior. Finally, given that one of the primary settings for developing socially in the LGB community is through bars and clubs, abstinence (while appropriate in some respects) may lead to social isolation. Individuals who can learn moderation and live a balanced life, decreasing the potential harm from substance use, can remain socially connected. Certainly, going to clubs and bars does not require one to drink at all, nor does it require one to engage in use of drugs such as methamphetamine. Illness models of substance abuse may lead to beliefs that a person cannot be exposed to high-risk situations without succumbing to pressure to drink or use drugs. Harm reduction and relapse prevention may prove to be effective means for teaching individuals how to maintain self-control in a variety of situations.

Chapter 8

Emerging Behavioral and Cognitive-Behavioral Therapies[1]

Behavior therapy is not a static methodology that does not change. Because so great an emphasis is placed on empirical study, innovative techniques and ideas are developed all of the time. This was surely the case when behavior therapy incorporated cognitive approaches. The philosophical dialogue among behavior analytic schools of thought, behavior therapy or social learning approaches, and cognitive approaches has added richness to the field, advancing it far beyond early behavior modification interventions with overt behavioral problems. This chapter provides brief discussions of five therapies that have emerged in the CBT arena. These five therapies—dialectical behavior therapy (DBT; Linehan, 1993a), acceptance and commitment therapy (ACT; Hayes et al., 1999), constructivist psychotherapy (Neimeyer & Mahoney, 1995), functional analytic psychotherapy (FAP; Kohlenberg & Tsai, 1991), and mindfulness-based cognitive therapy (Segal, Williams, & Teasdale, 2002)—share common features as well as providing unique interventions.

DIALECTICAL BEHAVIOR THERAPY

DBT (Linehan, 1993a) has been used with a variety problems, particularly in the treatment of women with borderline personality disorder (BPD), and presents a uniquely behavioral approach to the treatment of DSM-IV Axis II disorders. DBT was the first empirically supported treatment for chronically parasuicidal outpatients diagnosed BPD (Koerner

& Dimeff, 2000; Miller & Rathus, 2000). DBT is based on the philosophy of dialectics (Basseches, 1984), in which reality is seen to be in a state of continuous change, and truth evolves over time. Such a view of the world does not accept truth as absolute, and the philosophy accounts for opposing internal forces that remain in tension. In DBT the main dialectic is between acceptance and change. The DBT, therapist accepts the client exactly as she (or he) is, while also helping him or her to change self-destructive behaviors. DBT therapists balance tension between a variety of opposites, both challenging and nurturing a client, always considering the alternatives to the client's fixed beliefs (Linehan, 1993a). DBT is delivered with the use of multiple modalities. Clients involved in DBT for BPD work individually with a primary therapist but also participate in DBT skills training (Linehan, 1993b) group with a separate therapist. Thus, the patient in DBT works with a team of therapists rather than just one-on-one.

DBT is a theory, rather than a protocol driven therapy. However, therapists attend to a hierarchy of target behaviors determined according to the degree that the behaviors threaten the client and therapy. The order of target behaviors in the hierarchy is as follows, from highest to lowest priority:

1. Decreasing life-threatening, homicidal, suicidal, or parasuicidal behaviors.
2. Decreasing behaviors that interfere with treatment, such as non-compliance or dropout.
3. Decreasing behaviors that severely affect quality of life.
4. Increasing behavioral skills, such as emotion regulation, interpersonal skills, and problem solving.

All suicidal or parasuicidal behavior is top priority for a session agenda. The therapist works with the client to conduct a chain analysis of the situations and behaviors that led to the parasuicidal act or the suicidal ideation. DBT places a strong emphasis on fully orienting clients to the structure and rationale for the treatment (Amy Wagner, personal communication, October 31, 2002) to get them fully involved and committed to the process from the start.

With these difficult clients, much of the therapy may focus on prevention of harm. Linehan (1999, as cited in Miller & Rathus, 2000) has identified four aspects of BPD to be considered as treatment targets: (1) severe behavioral dyscontrol; (2) quiet desperation; (3) problems in living; and (4) incompleteness. The treatment development and research on DBT has primarily focused on the first target. When clients experience lives filled with chronic crisis, they must first learn to regulate their emotional responses before they can learn to live a more complete life.

There are many components to DBT. To date, research on DBT has only evaluated the treatment as a whole. It is not yet known whether the entire treatment approach is necessary, or whether skills training alone, or, for that matter, individual therapy alone, would be equally effective. Research has demonstrated that DBT is superior to treatment as usual in reducing the number and lethality of parasuicidal episodes, reducing psychiatric admissions, reducing anger, and improving overall functioning in women diagnosed with BPD (Linehan, Armstrong, Suarez, Allmon, & Heard, 1991; Turner, 2000).

DBT, originally developed for treating chronic suicidality, and later for treatment of clients meeting criteria for BPD, has now been expanded to treat other problems. Rathus and Miller (2000) modified DBT to treat suicidal adolescents and their families. DBT has also been used in the treatment of domestic violence (Fruzzetti & Levensky, 2000) and in a criminal justice setting with inpatient forensic clients (McCann, Ball, & Ivanoff, 2000). It has also been modified to treat women with BPD who are substance abusers (Dimeff, Rizvi, Brown, & Linehan, 2000) and even depressed elderly persons (Lynch, 2000). Linehan (2000) pointed out that the modifications to DBT for other populations relate to the classes of behaviors that must be eliminated or reduced, to skillful behaviors that must be increased, and to classes of behavior that are secondary targets, because they are functionally linked to the client's problem behaviors.

It is unlikely that DBT would need to be modified significantly for use with LGB clients. Therapists working with LGB clients diagnosed with BPD would target the same behaviors as those in working with heterosexual clients. Because large-scale treatment trials rarely include questions about sexual orientation in demographic data, it is hard to know how many LGB clients participate in such studies. Fortunately, most studies do not discriminate against LGB clients either (with the exception of some studies of couple therapy that exclude same-gender couples); there is, therefore, no reason to believe that the treatments would not generalize to the LGB population.

Dennis, a gay man who rejected many traditional norms of male behavior, was very expressive with his emotions. He dressed in bright colors and chose to wear leather more often than cotton. Dennis was prone to hyperbole and exaggeration as a method of being entertaining. He did not discriminate well between occasions that called for seriousness and those in which it was more appropriate to use camp humor, and he used such humor in his therapy sessions. Currently in his middle 50s, Dennis has been in therapy periodically since his early 30s. He

was misdiagnosed with a mixed personality disorder by his first therapist, who considered him to have features of both borderline and histrionic personality disorder. However, Dennis did not have a history of
parasuicidal behaviors. He had only begun dating men at age 30; hence,
he had not been in a long-term, meaningful relationship by the time of
his first therapeutic experience. He knew that he was not interested in
women sexually but had many close women friends, with whom he
maintained deeply loving friendships since high school. His relationships were neither intense nor unstable.

Dennis expressed suicidal ideation when he first saw his therapist,
following termination from a job in retail, under conditions that were
later shown to be discriminatory based on his sexual orientation and
gender-atypical behavior. When he first entered therapy, he had been
unemployed for 3 months, and his loss of a job triggered negative beliefs about self. People had repeatedly told him to "act like a man" and
not be so "girlie" when he was a teenager, and he had tried to mimic a
more masculine demeanor, until he decided to be true to himself, start
dating men, and get involved with the gay community. Once he felt that
he was a part of the gay community, he allowed himself to wear the
types of clothing he enjoyed rather than those he believed he was required to wear by societal standards. His first therapist (a heterosexual
male) thought that Dennis "flaunted" his sexuality, had an unstable
self-image, was sexually impulsive (based on the fact that Dennis had
begun to have sex once or twice a month at a local bathhouse), and had
chronic feelings of emptiness, because he stated that life felt meaning-
less, since he was uncertain about his career path. Dennis believed that
this therapist was not helpful; he pressured Dennis to be more "manly,"
in the same way that others had done throughout his life. He found a
second therapist—a heterosexual woman—who properly diagnosed
him—adjustment disorder with depressed mood—and focused on career counseling and disputing negative beliefs about himself. As a result
of the second therapy, Dennis explored career options that allowed him
to feel safe expressing himself in the fashion that he chose. He went
back to school to study fashion design and subsequently worked successfully as a costume designer in the theater. The diagnosis of borderline features and histrionic personality disorder were based on the stereotypical beliefs about appropriate male dress and demeanor that had
biased his original therapist. BPD is also often used as a catchall label
for difficult clients, or for those who are not successful in treatment.
Therapists must therefore take care to make the diagnosis properly, and
DBT is the behavioral treatment of choice for clients who do indeed
meet criteria for BPD.

Amelia, a 23-year-old, bisexual woman, entered outpatient therapy after being released from the hospital for a near-fatal suicide attempt. She had slashed both her wrists and ingested two bottles of Tylenol. She made her suicide attempt 30 minutes before an appointment with her girlfriend, Rhonda, to have a conversation about breaking up. Amelia had been cutting her arms and legs with razors since she was 12. She had been hospitalized twice before for suicidal gestures. She did have an unstable sense of self, but this was indicated not by her bisexuality, but by the persistent belief that she would "cease to exist" without a meaningful love relationship. Hence, she became intensely committed to both men and women after one or two dates and, typically, overwhelmed potential partners by declaring love and devotion before the relationship could truly develop. Whenever she sensed that a particular man or woman was about to end a relationship with her, Amelia would become hypersexual, meeting people on the Internet or at bars and desperately searching for a replacement. Her relationship with Rhonda had lasted longer than most—2 months. However, prior to her suicide attempt, Amelia had accused Rhonda of looking at other women and being unfaithful. When Rhonda told her that she did not believe they had talked about an exclusivity commitment, Amelia became enraged, called her an "insensitive slut," and told Rhonda that she wanted to "cut out her eyes and set her hair on fire." She then proceeded to punch herself in the forehead and say, "You've ripped out my heart, you bitch. You've ripped out my heart!" Rhonda left this encounter, telling Amelia that she was not going to tolerate such abuse. She only agreed to meet with Amelia to discuss breaking up after Amelia had pleaded with her not to end the relationship without closure. Thus, the date was planned, and Rhonda found Amelia in a tub of warm, bloody water.

Amelia was referred to a DBT therapist and attended a skills training group. Her therapy focused on decreasing self-harming behaviors. She wanted to improve her social skills so that she wouldn't scare off potential partners, but her therapist believed this desire actually functioned to maintain Amelia's dependence on others and the terror of being alone. Thus, Amelia's therapist made a contract with her to discuss her social life only after she had learned better coping skills than the parasuicidal behaviors in which she so frequently engaged. She was also referred to a second therapist's skills training group.

DBT was a pioneering attempt to include acceptance as a component in cognitive-behavioral treatment. Many people new to CBT regard it as treatment that focuses on changing behavioral or cognitive symptoms. Although change has been a primary focus, since it's inception, CBT has targeted emotional avoidance. Consider the treatment of anxiety disorders, PTSD, and OCD discussed earlier. The treatments all require clients to face situations they have avoided out of fear or distress, and to stay in the situation until their distress is reduced. CBT has frequently taught clients to act constructively in spite of their negative feelings. DBT took acceptance a step further, with the idea of "radical acceptance" (Linehan, 1993a) by the therapist for the client, and by the client for him- or herself. Since that time, other behavior therapies also have begun to create a balance between acceptance and change. Integrative behavioral couple therapy (see Chapter 6), for example, requires therapists to create an environment in which partners can talk about problems in a manner that encourages acceptance of the other. These newer behavior therapies account for the problem in which attempts to change oneself or one's partner, or to resist negative behaviors, ironically, often lead to worsening of the behavior rather than the desired change. Nowhere is this more clearly delineated than in acceptance and commitment therapy.

ACCEPTANCE AND COMMITMENT THERAPY

Acceptance and commitment therapy, ACT [pronounced "act"] (Hayes, Strosahl, & Wilson, 1999), offers the perspective of a radical behavioral formulation of verbal behavior that views avoidance of painful feelings as being at the heart of much psychological distress. ACT therapy emphasizes acceptance of thoughts and feelings as products of one's personal history rather than as truths that clients endorse. ACT also encourages clients to commit to behavior that is consistent with their values. It is based on complicated philosophical and behavioral concepts that are beyond the scope of this brief review. However, it is important that one understand how ACT departs from other cognitive and behavioral therapies on two basic issues: a philosophical worldview and an understanding of human cognition.

The philosophical core of ACT is functional contextualism (Hayes, 1993), which is arguably the philosophical basis of behavior analysis (Hayes, Hayes, & Reese, 1988). According to this philosophy, all acts are acts in context, and one part cannot be separated out into units without losing the whole. For example, fingers did not write the words on this page; rather, an entire action of writing occurred. Writing this page only makes sense when the whole process is taken into account. All behavior is contextually based, which means that nothing occurs in isolation, nor does anything have meaning apart from the context in which it occurs. Truth, according to contextualist philosophy, is defined as "what works," and this pragmatic truth criterion (Pepper, 1942) defines ACT. ACT therapists encourage clients to "stay with the experience of what works or does not work" (Hayes et al., 1999, p. 20).

When one speaks of changing context, an image of changing jobs or moving to a new city may come to mind. However, contextualists, particularly behavior analysts, are speaking of something else. When the ACT therapists speak of changing context, they are referring primarily to changing the social–verbal contexts that give verbal relations their functions. Verbal relations in human beings are fundamental. Nonhuman organisms can readily be trained in specific, unidirectional relations. When the organism is shown the color red (A) and rewarded when choosing an oval shape (B), then again is shown the color red and rewarded when it chooses a scratchy piece of sandpaper (C), the non-human organism can learn this task quite well and will over time pick either the oval shape (B) or the piece of sandpaper (C) when presented with the color red (A). In other words the organism has learned that A = B, and A = C. The human, however, derives a set of bidirectional relations when given the same unidirectional training. A human child given this training would be able to select red given ovals, or red given sandpaper, or sandpaper given ovals, or ovals given sandpaper. These kinds of "relational frames" (Hayes, Barnes-Holmes, & Roche, 2001) occur even in human infants, but slowly or not at all in nonhumans. Relational frames are central to human language.[2]

All of this is important, because events can take on stimulus properties of other events, based on the bidirectional relations between them. For example words such as "shock," "death," and "sick" themselves take on aversive properties, because they have been related to aversive events. If one hears the word "sick" each time he or she feels nauseous or feverish, over time, the word itself can elicit aversive properties of nausea or feeling flushed. Imagine having the experience of feeling slightly achy and tired, then saying, "I think I'm sick." Often telling oneself, "I think I'm sick," increases the feelings of achiness and fatigue. This is as true when one is actually suffering from an illness as when one merely has a nonspecific ache. When a client describes a negative interaction with her mother regarding a plan to have a baby via artificial insemination and raise the child with her female partner, and becomes tearful and upset in telling the story, this same process is occurring. The words used to tell the story, the memories, and so on, have taken on the same function as the original act. Thus, telling the story is an emotionally evocative process.

Undermining the typical impact of human language is at the heart of ACT. Because of the bidirectionality of human language, "it is aversive to be verbally aware of aversive events. Thus, avoidance of aversive private experiences is the natural result of human language" (Hayes et al., 1999, p. 45). An example of an "aversive private event" might be thinking about a breakup with a lover. The problem with trying to avoid such events deliberately is that to deliberately do something involves following a verbal rule. A verbal rule such as "do not think about the breakup'" will itself lead to thoughts of the breakup, because of the bidirectional relationship between the rule and the thought the person wants to avoid. ACT tries to break through this kind of self-amplifying process by challenging the need to control private events, by encouraging acceptance of and exposure to them, and by "deliteralizing" language (S. Hayes, personal communication, November 1, 2002). "Deliteralizing" language involves techniques that encourage clients to see thoughts merely as well-trained words related to other events rather than the actual presence of these other, related events. For example, a client might be asked to reduce a worrisome thought to a single word, then say that word over and over again, until it loses all meaning; or a client might be asked to practice "just noticing" troublesome thoughts, much as one does in meditation, rather than believing or disbelieving them. A wide variety of metaphors and exercises are used to teach clients not to "buy into" their thinking, or to avoid their various feelings. One can have the thought "I am feeling scared" and not "buy into" that thought, but simply accept it as one's brain chattering away. The thought, "I am feeling scared," need not be avoided, and no change in behavior "private or public" is necessary to make it go away. It is just a thought.

An acronym for the ACT approach to psychopathology is FEAR (Hayes, 2002; Hayes et al., 1999): fusion, evaluation, avoidance, and reason giving. *Fusion* refers to the process by which behavior becomes more verbally regulated and less sensitive to direct experience. In ACT language, derived functions dominate direct ones (Hayes, 2002, p. 59). A young man called a "faggot" throughout high school, for example, may avoid walking near groups of adolescent males because seeing the group and remembering his negative experience make him feel fear, even if there are no threat cues in the immediate situation, say, a group of adolescents playing pinball at an arcade. The process of *evaluation* increases human suffering, because human beings can compare their experience to events that they fear and wish to avoid, or that they wish to attain. A young law student, for example, who has been accepted into a law program at a major state university can feel discouraged and depressed because she was not accepted to an Ivy League school. The young man avoiding the group of adolescent boys at an arcade is an example of experiential *avoidance*, another of the main targets of ACT. Experiential avoidance is an unwillingness to remain in contact with an aversive private experience, such as a negative feeling, uncomfortable bodily sensation, and so on, and the subsequent steps the individual takes to escape or avoid the experience. Hayes (2002) suggests that the more negative private events are avoided, the more they occur, because the act of avoiding them reminds the individual of the events evoking the emotion to be avoided. We can take an example of coming out, which, admittedly, entails a broad class of behaviors, but helps to make a point about experiential avoidance. Imagine a young gay man who fears telling his father about his sexual orientation. When he thinks about coming out to his father, he feels anxious and worries about his father's response. He may imagine a negative interaction. Subsequently, he withholds details of his life from his father and becomes increasingly withdrawn from family events. His fear of being rejected, and the avoidance of aversive private events, actually make him feel badly and cause a disruption in his relationship with his father. His father's actual reaction may, indeed, be negative, and coming out to his father may in fact be painful for the young man. However, to avoid coming out is already painful and may create the very problem that the young man avoids, without the possibility of a different outcome.

ACT also seeks to undermine *reason giving*. People seek reasons for their behavior. The field of psychotherapy has promoted reason giving. When clients look to past events in their lives to explain something that causes them current distress, they construct a story about the past. For example, it might be concluded that Mary is having difficulty being emotionally intimate in her relationship with Judith, because an uncle sexually abused her when she was a young girl. The facts in this statement may be true, but they ignore myriad features that would be necessary to understand *why* the sexual abuse impacted Mary in precisely that way. If reason giving were useful, no one could object, but often the stories clients tell explain but do not improve their lives. Indeed, clients can often become more interested in being right about the reasons for their misery than about changing their own lives. Many of the reasons clients generate point to unchangeable events (e.g., a history of sexual abuse), and if reasons, literally, are causes, this means that the causes are also unchangeable. ACT tries to cut to the bottom line of actual behavior change. Reasons are just thoughts. Whatever "caused" the client's misery, the task now is to move ahead toward a more valued life.

One of the goals of ACT, therefore, is to help clients to live lives that they value, and to take action toward valued goals rather than to avoid aversive private experience. ACT therapists help clients to clarify values, to break experiential avoidance, through acceptance and willingness. The ACT client also must expose him- or herself to troublesome thinking, feelings, or bodily sensations. Although philosophically quite different from traditional cognitive therapy, the process of cognitive diffusion places ACT in the realm of cognitive therapy in helping clients to deliteralize language. Teaching clients to act rather than avoid troublesome experience is exposure, which is in keeping with traditional behavior therapies.

ACT has received support as an efficacious treatment in several outcome studies and single-case studies, although large-scale studies of treatment efficacy have not been published to date. Act has been used successfully in the treatment of depression (Zettle & Raines, 1989). In a field effective study at a large health maintenance organization (HMO) in the Northwest, master's-level therapists were given extensive ACT training. Compared to those not trained in ACT, the ACT therapists made fewer referrals for medication. Moreover, their clients were more likely to have completed therapy at 5-month assessment than the clients of the untrained therapists (Strosahl, Hayes, Bergan, & Romano, 1998).

COGNITIVE CONSTRUCTIVISM

Another variation on the theme of traditional cognitive-behavioral therapy is cognitive constructivism (Mahoney, 1995). Like ACT, cognitive constructivism is a contextual therapy. Unlike ACT, it does not rely on principles of behavior analysis or an understanding of verbal behavior in its conceptualization. Constructivist conceptualizations recognize that human beings receive feedback from and respond to their environment, as in traditional cognitive therapy formulations. Perceptions are important. However, constructivists also emphasize that people project their perceptions onto their environment. Such "feed forward" activity changes the environment in a reciprocal way, as the person receives feedback from the environment, thus changing him or her. Reality is therefore actively constructed. According to Mahoney (1995) constructivist therapies and rationalist cognitive therapies differ in three major ways. Rationalist therapies assume that (1) irrationality is the primary source of psychopathology, (2) beliefs can guide emotions and behavioral actions, and (3) effective psychotherapy substitutes rational for irrational thinking patterns (p. 8). Rationalist metatheory assumes that there is an objective, external reality that can be known, and that determines what is rational or irrational. In contrast, constructivist metatheory (1) adopts a proactive rather than a representational view of cognition, (2) emphasizes tacit (out of awareness) core ordering processes, and (3) "promotes a complex systems model in which thought, feeling, and behavior are interdependent expressions of a life span developmental unfolding of interactions between self and (primarily social) systems" (p. 8). The only reality that we can know for certain, therefore, is what is not (Watzlawick, 1996).

Psychotherapy, in cognitive constructivism, has been summarized nicely by Watzlawick (1996) as "the art of replacing a reality construction that no longer 'fits' with another, better-fitting one" (p. 68). This concept of reality shares the idea of truth as "what works" with contextualist thinking. This is a radical departure from traditional cognitive therapy. Although both traditional cognitive and constructivist therapies emphasize changing how the client perceives the world, the former does so by using reasoned discussion, teaching clients to look for empirical evidence to prove or disprove their beliefs, whereas the latter does not assume that the client will ever see the world as it really is, because there is no objective reality. Not all constructivist therapists believe they have made a radical departure from traditional cognitive therapy (Rosen & Kuehlwein, 1996). Rather, they recognize a tendency in Beckian cognitive therapy to be constructive in nature by avoiding emphasis on an external reality and having clients predict what will happen as a result of certain behaviors or beliefs (K. T. Kuehlwein, personal communication, October 28, 2002).

Constructivism, furthermore, does not accept a permanent self. Such a self is a constructed illusion that one holds through the narrative that has developed in the many transactions within a social community. Constructivist therapy is therefore centered on narrative, and changing narratives. This new development may be of particular interest to therapists working from a feminist perspective. We spoke earlier (Chapter 1) of the social constructionist view of the world as it relates to sexual orientation. Narratives about sexual orientation are socially constructed and differ from culture to culture and epoch to epoch, even if the physiological sensations experienced by human beings are relatively the same. Sexual attraction to a person of one sex or another is constructed differently and holds a different meaning. Sexual orientation as part of self-identity may be a relatively new construct, although same-sex sexual feelings have existed for as long as recorded history.

A constructivist approach may prove particularly useful when working with lesbian or bisexual women clients, who are more likely to regard their sexual orientation as a social construct. It is consistent with feminist approaches to psychotherapy (e.g., Brown, 1994) that make use of narrative. Delilah, a bisexual woman, was helped in therapy to change a narrative about herself as sexually confused and indecisive to seeing herself as open to loving many people. She began to define her sexual orientation as being attracted to "intelligent, gentle, and interpersonally engaging people" rather than to a particular gender, and she accepted that she found people who were slightly larger than average more physically attractive. She stopped defining herself by her sexual orientation and felt freer to date men and women who interested her without feeling that she was "a lesbian this month and a straight woman the next." She also became more open to having a long-term relationship with someone regardless of his or her gender.

FUNCTIONAL ANALYTIC PSYCHOTHERAPY AND ENHANCED COGNITIVE THERAPY

CBT has been stereotyped by some as highly technical and impersonal. In reality, a good therapeutic relationship is essential in CBT. Safran and Segal (1990) emphasized the importance of interpersonal processes in cognitive therapy and demonstrated that the relationship between client and therapist provides opportunities for clients to understand and test their beliefs about themselves and others.

Functional analytic psychotherapy (FAP; Kohlenberg & Tsai, 1991) provides a behavioral emphasis on the therapeutic relationship. It represents another in the newer innovations of behavior therapy. FAP is based on the premise that "the most clinically significant improvements in therapy are the result of evoking, prompting, shaping, and naturally reinforcing changes in the client's daily-life problematic behavior . . . that also occur in the session (Kohlenberg & Tsai, 1993, p. 81)." Based on Skinner's behavior analytic understanding of verbal behavior (1957), FAP recognizes that the function of the client's verbal behavior may be disguised in some way. Skinner broke verbal behavior into component parts such as "tacts," "mands," "intraverbals," and "autoclitics." We restrict our discussion of verbal behavior as it relates to FAP to tacts and mands, and the interested reader is referred to the original work (Skinner, 1957) for a more detailed analysis. Tacting is a relationship in which an object or event is a discriminative stimulus that sets the occasion for a particular verbal utterance. The statement, "I am wearing red shoes," is a tact, because the object, "red shoes," has set the occasion for the utterance. In the language of radical behaviorism, a client who says (overtly or covertly), "I am a worthless piece of worthlessness" may simply be tacting his or her experience of repeated failures and disappointments. "Mands" are verbal responses that specify a consequence, such as making a request or a command. Hence, the statement, "Bring me a glass of water," is a mand, as is the statement, "I would like a glass of water," because in both cases, receiving a glass of water is the specified consequence of the utterance.

Sometimes statements that appear to be tacts are actually disguised mands. Take the example in the last paragraph of the client who says, "I am a worthless piece of worthlessness." What appears to be a client tacting his or her experience may in fact turn out to be a disguised mand, if the client is trying to obtain sympathy, support, or help. How would the therapist know that this is the case? According to Kohlenberg and Tsai (1991), the therapeutic relationship provides the key. FAP therapists are taught to look for three types of clinically relevant behaviors (CRBs). CRB1 is problem behavior that occurs during the therapy session. CRB2 is any improvement in the client's behavior. FAP therapists want to reinforce CRB2. In CRB3, the client demonstrates understanding between his or her behavior and its consequences. Therapists should look for CRB1 and ask careful questions that may evoke CRB1—such as "What is your reaction to what I just said?"— and reinforce CRB2 and CRB3. Take the following dialogue with the client who states, "I am a worthless piece of worthlessness" as an example:

CLIENT: I've been feeling very badly about myself lately [a tact, possibly a disguised mand].

THERAPIST: Has this been worse during the past week than in previous weeks?

CLIENT: I just don't know. I'm just a worthless piece of worthlessness in my mind [CRB1, possibly a disguised mand].

THERAPIST: Do you think you are a worthless piece of worthlessness when you are here with me? [Probes to see whether the statement has another meaning, whether it is functioning as a hidden mand.]

CLIENT: Well, I guess so. I worry that you don't care about me. Why should you? I'm just another gay guy with HIV to you. [More CRB1, but the therapist would accept that the client is moving in the right direction and try to shape the behavior further.]

THERAPIST: I think that I should care about you because you are my client, because we have a relationship, and I enjoy being in your company.

CLIENT: Yeah, but you have a lot of clients, and I bet you care about them all. Your other clients didn't screw up their lives by barebacking[3] with some jerk who was doing everyone in town.

THERAPIST: How does thinking that I have other clients, or that you've screwed up your life, relate to your worrying that I don't care about you?

CLIENT: I don't know. You probably don't care about me in particular.

THERAPIST: [not wanting to reinforce CRB1] How could you recognize whether I care or not?

CLIENT: I should be able to tell, but I'm too fucked up. I guess I could ask you if you care, but that would be stupid.

THERAPIST: What makes you say "that would be stupid"?

CLIENT: It just sounds so pathetic.

THERAPIST: If I do, in fact, care about you, what harm would there be in asking me?

CLIENT: But if you don't really care, I'd sound like even more of an idiot.

THERAPIST: Yes, I see your point. It is a bit of a risk, isn't it? So when you told me that you thought you were a worthless piece of worthlessness, was there anything else you were trying to tell me?

CLIENT: I guess I was hoping you'd tell me that I wasn't one [getting closer to the target of directly asking the therapist].

THERAPIST: I understand. You wanted to hear that I care about you [trying to shape the client's behavior to asking a direct question]. That seems like a legitimate desire. If I were you, I'd want to trust that my therapist cared about me and thought I was worthwhile. I'd also want to know that my therapist doesn't think that I'm a screw up, or judge me.

CLIENT: Well, do you? [CRB2; the typically unassertive client asks the therapist directly.]

THERAPIST: No, I don't think you are a screw up. And yes, I care about you very much. It makes me feel a little sad for you that you have been feeling so badly this past week. I also think that you made the sexual choices you did because you trusted [his ex] to be telling you the truth when he said the two of you were monogamous [responding naturally to the question, thus reinforcing CRB2].

CLIENT: I guess I don't ever really ask what people think about me. I just try to beat around the bush to see what people might do. That probably makes me feel worse. [CRB3; the client makes a connection between his unassertive behavior and feeling worse.]

THERAPIST: How did it feel just now to ask me?

CLIENT: Scary.

THERAPIST: How does it feel to know that I care about you and understand that you didn't intentionally become HIV-positive?

CLIENT: Good, I feel a little better. I know you are my therapist and are supposed to care and be nonjudgmental [CRB1], but it at least helps me to know that somebody does.

   The reader by now should have a feel for how a typical CBT session might go and may recognize the difference between the preceding FAP interchange and what may occur more typically in CBT. Therapists trained in traditional CBT might look at the thought, "I'm a worthless piece of worthlessness," as either an automatic thought or a core belief, then assist the client in looking for evidence to support or refute the belief, and try to shake the client's rigid adherence to such an absolute label. The FAP therapist did not question the client's statement, but instead probed to uncover the function of the statement. In this case, the statement functioned as a request for reassurance from the therapist. Rather than simply say, "OK, now I know that your statement really means that you are asking me if I care about you," the therapist worked with the client to exhibit an improvement on the nonassertive behavior by ultimately asking directly, "Do you care?"

   Although the radical behavioral conceptualization in FAP differs from a cognitive conceptualization, FAP is not inconsistent with cognitive therapy. In fact, Kohlenberg and Tsai (1994), suggested that adding FAP principles to cognitive therapy could enhance cognitive therapy by adding a focus on the therapeutic relationship. Kohlenberg, Kanter, Bolling, Parker, and Tsai (2002) added FAP to cognitive therapy in an approach they referred to as FAP-enhanced cognitive therapy (FECT). In an FECT approach, the therapist focuses on in-session behaviors (CRBs) as in FAP, with a special emphasis on dysfunctional cognition as it relates to the therapeutic relationship. FECT therapists make use of the moment, trying to recognize CRB1 when it occurs in the form of negative thoughts regarding the therapist, the client in relation to the therapist, or the client as he or she is feeling in the session. This method of using the therapeutic relationship as the primary means to change makes use of variables that are somewhat in the control of the therapist. Clients can be given immediate feedback about the therapist's true thoughts or feelings. Even if the therapist is thinking negatively about a client, the relationship can be used to benefit the client in negotiating interpersonal difficulties or containing negative responses. The following is an example:

CLIENT: I know I shouldn't have told Tania to leave, and that getting really drunk afterward was just a cowardly way out.

THERAPIST: You responded to finding out that Tania had used your credit card number to make a purchase online, and you were angry. Were you acting out of anger?

CLIENT: Of course, I was acting out of anger. What a stupid question. She used my card and spent my money! Anybody would be angry.

Wouldn't you? That's my private property! Do you like it when people take advantage of you?

THERAPIST: It sounds like you are angry with me for asking that question.

CLIENT: Well, I am just angry in general. You are my therapist, and you're supposed to deal with it when I'm angry.

THERAPIST: Well, I actually feel uncomfortable when you get angry as quickly as you did just now. I understand how quickly it can happen, but also wonder if there are times that you say things or do things that you later regret? I think you aren't angry at me, necessarily, but simply angry at the situation, so you're more easily annoyed. Is that right?

CLIENT: Yes, I'm not really angry with you. I am annoyed. I also am feeling like I acted too quickly by telling Tania to leave. It isn't the worst offense in the world. I've let her use my credit card in the past, and I gave her the number. I didn't give her a chance to explain herself, and just kicked her out, then tried to calm myself with alcohol.

THERAPIST: So perhaps you regret acting prematurely on your feeling about Tania, just like you acted on the feeling of annoyance with me. Shall we try to work on difficulty that you have keeping yourself from reacting so fast when you are upset?

CLIENT: Yes, that would be good.

A small clinical trial comparing traditional cognitive therapy to FECT (Kohlenberg et al., 2002) has demonstrated several differences between the two therapies. Therapists conducting FECT did indeed focus more on the therapeutic relationship than when they conducted traditional cognitive therapy. Ironically, however, there were few examples of the same FECT therapists focusing on in-session cognition. This study was a treatment development study, and therapist competence in conducting FECT improved over time. Further research is needed to assess whether the additions to traditional cognitive therapy offered by FECT improve on the well-established efficacy of cognitive therapy for depression.

MINDFULNESS-BASED COGNITIVE THERAPY FOR DEPRESSION

Another modification of cognitive therapy has been developing in studies of relapse prevention for clients who have successfully completed cognitive therapy for depression. The new model teaches mindfulness as a strategy for preventing depression relapse. Mindfulness-based cognitive therapy (Segal et al., 2002) incorporates a number of features of some of the therapies discussed previously. Mindfulness is one of the core skills of DBT (Linehan, 1993b) and is taught as a means of helping clients to develop a greater capacity for acceptance of themselves and other people (Robins, 2002). Meditation has been a part of relapse prevention for substance abuse since its beginnings (Marlatt & Gordon, 1985; Marlatt, Pagano, Rose, & Marques, 1984). ACT (Hayes et al., 2000), like mindfulness-based cognitive therapy, seeks to break old patterns of thinking that are "driven by an overriding wish to get rid of the negative mood, and a strong attachment to the goal of feeling happy" (Segal et al., 2002, p. 91). ACT also recognizes the individual's desire to feel happy and thus avoid or escape negative affective experiences as problematic. The ACT therapist attempts to deliteralize language. In a similar way, mindfulness-based cognitive therapists teach clients that thoughts are just thoughts; that they do not need to be attended to, or acted upon, but that they can be watched nonjudgmentally and allowed to enter consciousness; furthermore, persons practicing mindfulness skills can bring themselves back to the object, situation, word, and so on, to which they are attending.

Mindfulness-based cognitive therapy provides a way to help depressed clients stop ruminating over their problems or bad circumstances. Nolen-Hoeksema, Morrow, & Fredrickson (1993) found that depressed clients who passively ruminated about their problems were more depressed for longer durations of time than those who took an active problem-solving approach. These findings have influenced various depression researchers to look at ruminations as targets for behavior change. This is the primary focus of mindfulness-based cognitive therapy, and has also been one of the treatment targets in behavioral activation treatment for depression (Martell et al., 2001).

Mindfulness-based cognitive therapy, as developed by Segal et al. (2002), is usually conducted in a group. It is an eight-session program for prevention of relapse. Each session teaches clients about specific mindfulness skills. Session 1 teaches the problems of living on "automatic pilot" or going through life without attending. In session 2, the therapist teaches clients how to deal with barriers they may encounter when practicing mindfulness. Session 3 teaches clients mindfulness of the breath, a frequent meditation practice. Session 4 teaches clients about "staying present" and becoming aware of their experiences, good or bad. Session 5 is specifically about acceptance and allowing negative feelings. In the sixth session, clients learn that thoughts are not facts, that thoughts are simply thoughts. As we pointed out earlier, this resembles the deliteralizing of ACT. Session 7 deals with self-care, and in the eighth session, clients are taught how to use their new skills in the future.

Mindfulness-based cognitive therapy is a relative newcomer in the ever-changing world of CBT. There is evidence that attention training (Wells, 1990), in which depressed clients are taught to focus attention away from themselves, is an effective technique in the treatment of recurrent major depression (Papageorgiou & Wells, 2001). Research from laboratories in California (e.g., Nolen-Hoeksema and colleagues), Canada (e.g., Segal), and England (e.g., Teasdale and colleagues, Wells and colleagues) have pointed out the importance of breaking patterns of rumination in the treatment of depression. This new focus in cognitive and behavioral practice holds promise for the future in preventing relapse in persons with chronic depression.

The models presented in this chapter represent the breadth of cognitive and behavioral treatments. Elements of these treatments have been a part of CBT for many years, and there is little that is radical about any of them. However, such is the movement of science and practice. Theories and ideas build on former knowledge and broaden in application. The new behavioral therapies are empirically based and do not represent a move away from the traditional CBT focus on science, or a move toward overemphasizing philosophy.

It is not clear how these new variations in cognitive and behavioral therapy will hold over time. Nor is it clear whether they will specifically benefit treatment with LGB adults. We offer the possibility, however, that balancing notions of acceptance and change (e.g., DBT, ACT), paying close attention to the therapeutic relationship (e.g., FAP, FECT), helping clients to understand constructions of their own realities through language (e.g., cognitive constructivism, ACT) and remaining present with experience (e.g., mindfulness) will help LGB clients who have a long history of distrust of change-oriented behavioral therapists. An emphasis on relationship and acceptance in CBT is an important step in providing affirmative therapy to diverse clients.

Chapter 9

Ethical Considerations and Clinical Judgment

Any therapist, of any sexual orientation, at some point works with clients who identify as LGB, or as members of a sexual minority group. As is the case in treating anyone from a minority culture, therapists are required to provide culturally competent and ethical treatment. Learning to do this requires training and experience. Being LGB alone does not qualify one to work with this population. Although the behavioral health professions treated LGB people as disordered for so many years, only in the last three decades has an affirmative approach to working with this population emerged. This is relatively new territory for the profession, and controversy continues for some about the acceptability of LGB and transgendered orientations and behaviors. Codes of ethics, standards of practice, and guidelines for care must allow intellectual, academic, and civil freedom for practitioners who hold a variety of viewpoints. However, the major behavioral health associations and organizations have begun to develop positions on appropriate therapeutic treatment with LGB clients that can inform clinicians of their ethical responsibilities and assist them in making sound clinical choices.

In this chapter, we discuss how ethical standards, principles, and clinical guidelines inform the practice of CBT with LGB clients. There are also issues of particular relevance to this population that require sound clinical judgment based on empirical findings, when the ethical codes and practice guidelines do not directly address the issue. First, we talk about the controversial practice of so-called conversion therapy, or reparative therapies, that attempt to change a person's sexual orienta-

191

tion. These practices are typically conducted by therapists and para-professionals espousing negatively biased views of LGB identities, often doing so on the basis of religious rather than scientific grounds.

For therapists who currently practice LGB-affirmative therapy, we address the issue of maintaining boundaries in therapy. This is particularly relevant to LGB therapists practicing with clients from a minority community, in which overlap between professional and personal lives may more frequently occur. Finally, we make several recommendations regarding ethical and clinically sound practice for CBT therapists working with LGB clients.

ETHICAL STANDARDS, PRINCIPLES, AND CLINICAL GUIDELINES

Ethical standards are enforceable codes of conduct. Violating an ethical standard can result in professional sanctions against a therapist. Ethical standards cannot be exhaustive, however. Therefore, conduct that is not specifically addressed in ethics codes can still be unethical, depending on the particular behavior and context. Ethical principles are aspirational, as are clinical guidelines; they provide the practitioner with the ideal to which he or she should strive. While not enforceable, principles and guidelines inform competent professional practice.

The *Ethical Principles of Psychologists and Code of Conduct* (American Psychological Association, 2002) provides several general principles, as well as specific standards, that are applicable when working with LGB clients. The ethical principles and code of conduct apply only to psychologists in their professional role; therefore, they do not dictate the behavior of psychologists in their personal lives. The American Psychological Association cannot require an individual who is a psychologist to be free from prejudice or bias in his or her personal life. However, Principle E states that when acting in their role as psychologists, they are

> aware of and respect cultural, individual, and role differences, including those based on age, gender, gender identity, race, ethnicity, culture, national origin, religion, sexual orientation, disability, language, and socioeconomic status and consider these factors when working with members of such groups. Psychologists try to eliminate the effect on their work of biases based on those factors. (p. 1063)

Because this is an ethical principle, and not a standard of conduct, it is aspirational. A psychologist who believes that LGB people are sinful, morally corrupt, or developmentally delayed cannot be sanctioned for holding such beliefs, nor would he or she be brought up on ethical violations if he or she stated such to clients. Some clients seek counseling from religiously oriented therapists, who may hold particular beliefs that might be considered biased against LGB people. Although clinical judgment may be questioned (we have more to say about this in the section on conversion therapy), unless another ethical standard is violated or there is documented harm to the client, the therapist is not acting unethically.

The National Association of Social Workers (1999) has gone further in its Code of Ethics. Not only does it state that social workers should respect the dignity and worth of each person, and understand the nature of social diversity, but also that they should "act to prevent and eliminate domination of, exploitation of, and discrimination against any person, group, or class on the basis of race, ethnicity, national origin, color, sex, sexual orientation, age, marital status, political belief, religion, or mental or physical disability" (p. 21). Although this is not expressly a call to political action, the terms "prevent" and "eliminate" imply some form of social activity. Once again, these are principles, not codes of conduct. The National Association of Social Workers is not dictating that members of their organization must be social activists.

When we say that these principles are aspirational, and that a member of one of these professional organizations is not acting unethically if he or she does not abide by these principles, we by no means intend to dilute the power of the principles. These aspirational principles are written into the ethical codes because they are seen as representing the highest standards of excellence for these professions. They also reflect the values held by the professions. These may not be the values held by individual members as private citizens, but, as professionals, such individuals should strive to uphold these principles.

A professional who holds biased or prejudicial views toward a particular group stands at a delicate precipice between maintaining his or her rights as a citizen and engaging in acts that would indeed constitute a breach of the standards of ethics, which are enforceable. For psychologists, the American Psychological Association's (2002) code of conduct has several standards that apply to working with diverse populations. A psychologist who bases decisions on theories that have been disproved or on which new data have cast doubt, or solely upon his or her own personal or religious beliefs may be in violation of the code of ethics. Ethical code 2.01(a) states that "psychologists provide services, teach, and conduct research with populations and in areas only within the boundaries of their competence." Standard 2.01(b) further states that "where scientific or professional knowledge in the discipline of psychology establishes that an understanding of factors associated with age, gender, gender identity, race, ethnicity, culture, national origin, religion, sexual orientation, disability, language, or socioeconomic status is essential for effective implementation of their surveys or research, psychologists have or obtain the training, experience, consultation, or supervision necessary to ensure the competence of their services" (American Psychological Association, 2002, pp. 4–5). The psychologist's work is to be based on established scientific and professional knowledge of the discipline (standard 2.04). A psychologist who believes that LGB individuals are developmentally delayed and treats LGB clients on the basis of that belief would be in violation of these codes of conduct, because the literature in the field has firmly established that LGB persons are not mentally ill or deviants. The literature suggesting that LGB people may have higher rates of specific psychological disorders such as anxiety and depression (discussed Chapters 4 and 5) also has concluded that the differences between rates of these disorders in LGB versus heterosexual samples is greatly reduced when the impact of discrimination experience is controlled.

One of the overarching ethical standards for all behavioral health practitioners is to "do no harm." Psychologists are thus to take reasonable steps to avoid harming their clients. This means obtaining informed consent when conducting any psychotherapeutic technique that has been shown to cause harm in some participants, and to provide alternative perspectives and treatments. This is true, of course, in general CBT practice as well. For example, when a therapist proposes a course of exposure therapy for PTSD, the potential client should be informed that the therapy may cause an increase in anxiety symptoms (see discussion, Chapter 7) and that there are several alternative approaches available to treat PTSD. Informed consent is also necessary when treating LGB adults (see the following discussion of conversion therapy). The need to obtain informed consent is specified in standards 3.10 and 10.01.

The three largest mental health organizations in the United States— the American Psychological Association, the American Psychiatric Association, and the National Association of Social Workers—all have policies and positions on working with sexual minority clients. The Association for Advancement of Behavior Therapy also has a fact sheet in press on cognitive behavioral therapy with LGB and transgender clients. Although guidelines are not necessarily enforceable, they provide an instructive blueprint for practitioners and evaluate their competence to work with this population.

On February 26, 2000, the American Psychological Association

(2000) adopted a set of guidelines for psychotherapy with LGB clients. Guidelines are not standards and cannot be enforced in the manner of ethical standards. However, the adoption of these guidelines has provided an initial step in assisting psychotherapists in making sound clinical judgment in treating LGB clients. The guidelines are separated into four sections, including "attitudes toward homosexuality and bisexuality," "relationships and family," "issues of diversity," and "education." There are 16 guidelines in all.

The guidelines are clear that there is no single LGB community. Individuals from all racial, ethnic, and cultural backgrounds may identify as LGB. Furthermore, definitions of LGB may differ from culture to culture, and psychologists must be sensitive to such differences. They should not only understand the particular challenges faced by lesbian and gay people of color but also those of bisexual individuals, LGB youth, and those with physical, sensory, cognitive, or emotional disabilities. The recognition of intergenerational differences in LGB communities is also encouraged.

The final section of the guidelines admonishes psychologists to support professional education regarding LGB issues and to obtain such training to increase their knowledge. Psychologists also must familiarize themselves with relevant community resources for their LGB clients.

ISSUES UNIQUE TO WORKING WITH LGB CLIENTS

Not all therapists who work with LGB individuals identify as such themselves. Many of the therapists and researchers working in this area of LGB mental health, however, do identify as LGB, and sharing this affinity with the LGB community may engender positive attitudes and an affirmative approach (Malyon, 1982; Perez, DeBord, & Bieschke, 2000) to the population. However, therapists of all sexual orientations must recognize that their opinions and personal experiences may strengthen but can, at times, also hinder competent and ethical practice. Two clinical issues unique to work with LGB clients are therapist disclosure of sexual orientation and the role of reparative or "conversion" therapies in working with LGB adults. LGB therapists working with this population may find that their professional and personal lives occasionally intersect. We therefore address the issue of multiple relationships. Therapists who are LGB, people of color, or who live in small, rural areas are frequently confronted with this third issue, because there is a greater possibility of connection with clients outside of the therapeutic setting as the breadth of one's community is narrowed.

Self-Disclosure

The question of whether clinicians should reveal details of their personal lives is rarely addressed in the ethical literature, but the issue is of key importance in working with LGB clients. In American culture, clients often assume that their therapist is heterosexual (Stein, 1988, cited in Hancock, 1995). In many contexts, clients enter therapy with the internalized anti-homosexual belief that heterosexuality is the norm, and that LGB people do not have mainstream careers—especially those that require advanced training. Certainly, as more LGB professionals are open about their sexual orientation, and as there are increasing numbers of openly LGB politicians and leaders, this misperception will diminish. However, in the meantime, LGB clients have two choices: search out specifically a therapist who is LGB or enter therapy not knowing a therapist's sexual orientation and hope that the therapist will at least be familiar with or practice LGB-affirmative psychotherapy.

Sexual orientation is not outwardly apparent. Unlike gender or race, a person's sexual orientation can remain hidden. Therapist gender, ethnicity, race, and other characteristics can all have an impact on therapy. Take, for example, a female client who has experienced men as distant, uncaring, and emotionally uninvolved. If she seeks therapy from a male therapist in the hope of working through issues about men, and finds a therapist who is empathic, connected, and emotionally present, her therapeutic experience will provide evidence to challenge her beliefs about men. This may be important for improving relationships with men in her family, colleagues at work, or potential romantic partners. Consider the following dialogue between a gay male client and his therapist:

GAY MALE CLIENT: All gay men suck. I just have not been able to have any type of relationship with gay men. They are all so superficial. Especially in this city, they are all so shallow and fake. I just think it's impossible to relate to any of them.

GAY MALE THERAPIST: Hmm . . . so let's see. Let's look at the evidence for what you are saying. You just made kind of a strong statement there—"I have not been able to have any type of relationship with gay men."

At this point, the gay male therapist has a perfect opportunity to use the therapeutic relationship as an example of a good relationship that the client has experienced. If the client does not know the therapist is gay, however, such an inference will be impossible for the client to draw. The therapist certainly can ask about other relationships, and it is quite likely that the absolute statement will be disproven by evidence from the client's life outside of therapy. Nevertheless, a potentially powerful, here-and-now intervention would be missed.

When LGB clients seek LGB therapists, they usually do so believing that such a therapist will better understand their experience. Many LGB clients seek LGB therapists because they fear that a heterosexually identified therapist will discriminate against them or consider their sexual orientation a problem. Some heterosexual therapists continue to attribute client problems per se to sexual orientation, even in the face of evidence that this is not the case (Garnets et al., 1991). When clients ask therapists about their sexual orientation, however, this is often interpreted as an invasion into the therapist's privacy. Traditional psychoanalytic notions of therapist neutrality have discouraged therapist self-disclosure on a number of issues. Regarding sexual orientation, however, even some psychoanalysts have encouraged therapists to be open with LGB clients (Isay, 1991). When a client asks about a particular therapist's sexual orientation, he or she is asking about a demographic factor that is not usually observable in the same manner as gender and race. Clients usually know that their therapist is male or female, for example. These are observable demographics; it is therefore justified for clients to ask whether their therapist is LGB, which is not so readily observed. Knowing that their therapist is LGB lessens clients' fear of judgment.

Therapists should, of course, use clinical judgment before disclosing in certain circumstances, and there may be clinical reasons for not doing so. For example, a sexually compulsive gay male client who is extremely seductive may have greater success in learning to develop an unsexualized relationship if he does not know the sexual orientation of his therapist. Typically, it is preferable for the therapist to be matter-of-fact about his or her orientation in the same way that therapists wear wedding rings, have pictures of spouses or children on their desks, or continue to go to work when they are pregnant. All of these examples of self-disclosures on the part of the therapist may become clinical issues in some cases (e.g., the need to discuss disruption of therapy following the birth of a child for a pregnant therapist) but mostly will be nonissues. We are in no way saying therapists must disclose. Rather, maintaining a rigid attitude about boundaries and privacy in this regard could be detrimental for LGB clients.

When a client knows his or her therapist is LGB, he or she can relate to the therapist as a role model in many ways. For clients who have not had experience with openly LGB professionals, the relationship with the therapist can be essential in understanding the diversity of roles that LGB people play. This may be particularly important for those working in rural areas, where access to the LGB community is restricted.

LGB clients need not see only LGB therapists. Many heterosexually identified therapists have appropriate training and experience to work with the LGB community. The same principle regarding disclosure would apply with heterosexually identified therapists; that is, if the client asks whether it is appropriate to disclose; if the client does not ask, it is not necessary to disclose. However, should the client make statements indicating that he or she assumes the therapist to be of a particular sexual orientation, the therapist can learn much by questioning the basis for the assumption. For example, a young gay man may tell a therapist that he assumed he was straight, because he "didn't act gay." There is a wealth of information in this one disclosure. The client is making assumptions about how gay people act, that a man who does not meet stereotypical images must be heterosexual, or that heterosexual men act in a certain manner. Also, the client may be expressing negative beliefs about himself, and the therapist would do well to be aware of future criticism made by the client regarding his own behaviors and mannerisms. Therefore, there are ethical and clinical reasons to take a flexible stance toward therapist self-disclosure when working with LGB clients.

Many LGB therapists advertise in LGB-affirmative publications or directories. Their sexual orientation is assumed by virtue of doing this. Non-LGB-identified therapists who also advertise their services to the LGB community may be presumed to be LGB. The same rule of thumb regarding disclosure should apply—if clients ask, tell; if they don't, there is not necessarily a need to do so. One caveat for the heterosexually identified therapist is to maintain a calm and neutral stance on disclosing sexual orientation when a client has assumed that he or she is LGB. By asking whether the therapist is LGB, an LGB client may be vulnerable to taking offense if the therapist is too quick to deny. In the following two hypothetical exchanges between client and therapist, the first is a less desirable response from the therapist, and the second, more desirable.

Less desirable:

CLIENT: I don't want to pry, but I called you because you were listed in the pink pages,[1] and I was wondering if you are gay?

THERAPIST: No, I'm not gay, but I've worked with gay and lesbian clients for years. [By this time, some clients may have already become emotionally distant. Historically, being made to feel shame and fear when incorrectly assuming someone to be gay or lesbian makes such an interaction a strong discriminative stimulus for further shame and guilt.]

   More desirable:

CLIENT: I don't want to pry, but I called you because you were listed in the pink pages, and I was wondering if you are gay?

THERAPIST: I'm glad you asked me, and glad you found me through the Pink Pages—I've advertised there for years. I completely understand if you'd rather work with a therapist who is gay, lesbian, or bisexual, but I identify as heterosexual. [Expressing validation for the possibility of the client preferring a different therapist confirms that the therapist does not claim privileged status due to being heterosexual. This response is collaborative and would be less likely to be misinterpreted as a judgment against the client for assuming that the therapist is gay.]

   It is inappropriate for therapists to make comments that can be interpreted as condescending or patronizing. Heterosexual therapists should never say things such as "I don't mind that people think I'm gay." Such a statement suggests that the therapist is particularly magnanimous toward being called by an undesirable name. Likewise, an LGB therapist should never be flippant, with a response such as "Do you have to ask?" This implies that the question is a joke and assumes too much familiarity with the client. Few therapists intentionally offend clients, but mistakes can be made in the name of making the client or the therapist feel comfortable. The stance that guarantees client comfort is usually a warm, supportive, and professional one.
   Not all therapists are supportive of homosexuality or bisexuality as normal variants of human sexual orientation (e.g., Nicolosi, 1991). Some practitioners who hold conservative religious viewpoints (e.g., Yarhouse & Burkett, 2002) argue that religious diversity must be respected in the same way as sexual-orientation diversity, and that for some conservative religious people, sexual orientation or sexual intimacy is not core to a sense of identity. Therefore, they argue that individuals seeking to change their sexual orientation on the basis of conservative religious views of the morality or immorality of homosexuality or bisexuality should be afforded treatment. Such a stance assumes the normality of heterosexuality and therefore justifies "treatment" of sexual orientation when clients are in conflict about their sexual orientation and their religious beliefs. This is truly a difficult issue that is not easily resolved by LGB-affirmative therapists (who cannot take a client's

religious beliefs lightly) or by anti-LGB therapists (who should not use the guise of being client-centered as a justification of heterosexist treatment).

Campos and Hathaway (1993) specifically have criticized behavior therapy for its lack of involvement in gay-related research beyond early attempts to change sexual orientation (see discussion of this issue in the Preface).[2] Therapists who believe it is necessary to provide therapy to LGB individuals wishing to change sexual orientation are in the minority, and conversion therapies are marginalized in mainstream psychology (Haldeman, 2002). We now briefly turn to another unique clinical–ethical issue in working with LGB adults.

"Conversion Therapy"

Those who support conversion therapy (also referred to as "sexual reorientation therapy" or "reparative therapy") say it is the ethical responsibility of practitioners to offer treatment to people seeking it (Yarhouse, 1998). Those opposed to conversion therapy point to the coercive nature of such therapy (from social pressure, mandates to therapy, in some cases, or pressure within the treatment that the only acceptable outcome is heterosexuality) and the lack of evidence that conversion therapy is actually helpful (Haldeman, 1994, 2002). Mainstream psychiatry, psychology, social work, and counseling associations have all considered sexual orientation to be varied, and this variation to be a normal part of human behavior. So-called reparative therapy, however, is practiced under the assumption that heterosexuality is the only normal sexual orientation, that changing a person's sexual behavior is a moral imperative, and that clients' lives will be better if they live according to heterosexual norms.

Haldeman (2002), acknowledging that there is an unresolved tension between respecting diversity in sexual orientation and in religious belief, addressed many of the problems inherent in conversion therapy. Results of studies of sexual reorientation or conversion suffer from bias in a number of areas. First and foremost, these studies are subject to sampling bias, and data on randomized samples do not exist. Second, the studies suffer from response bias, because the participants, researchers, therapists, and evaluators maintain social bias against homosexuality or bisexuality as a variant of normal sexual orientation and are highly motivated to demonstrate the success of conversion therapy as a valid treatment. Participants, furthermore, often seek treatment because they belong to conservative religious groups that denounce homosexuality and bisexuality, and are therefore highly motivated to change their orientation, or to claim that treatment was a success in spite of less clear outcome data. Drescher (2001) suggested that sexual conversion therapy demonstrates a lack of respect for patients' religious and cultural beliefs (being predominantly coercive regarding conservative religious and cultural views), that it is frequently harmful to patients, and that it promotes social conformity above and beyond the specific needs of the individual. CBT therapists need to be aware that a client's desire to change may be based on irrational beliefs about being LGB that have been learned in an invalidating environment (Purcell, Campos, & Perilla, 1996). For those who have had little exposure to LGB experience and may only know what is presented in the media or from the pulpit, or who have participated only in sexual aspects of LGB life, irrational ideas such as "I can never have a loving family if I'm gay or lesbian" or "Everyone will reject me if I am openly gay" may prevail.

Claims about successful change in restricted samples of primarily religious individuals who are highly motivated to conform to the conservative norms of their religious groups are spurious at best. The mostly anecdotal data suggest that some individuals improve on measures of depression and anxiety (Throckmorton, 2002). However, the resultant change in emotional distress in these clients may be due to reconciliation of religious beliefs. Certainly cognitive behavioral therapists and researchers, who have a long history of questioning research that uses self-report methods alone as dependent measures, must recognize the questionable outcomes of such methods. Research that reports "success" in treating people who initially believed their same-sex attractions were immoral, unnatural, and unwanted, and who, then, following treatment, report that they no longer have same-sex fantasies or attractions, is strongly subject to both experimenter and participant bias.

Shroeder and Shidlo (2001a) sought to understand better the experience of individuals treated with conversion therapy. They interviewed 150 consumers of sexual conversion therapies who had this treatment somewhere between 1995 and 2000. To be included in their study, participants needed to have a history of at least six conversion therapy sessions and a pretreatment self-report of 5–6 on the Kinsey scale (*mostly homosexual–exclusively homosexual*). The participants also were required to have been in therapy conducted by a licensed or certified mental health professional. Schroeder and Shidlo (2001b) asked participants about pretherapy disclosure by therapists. Only 26% of the time did clinicians inform the client that neither the American Psychiatric Association nor the American Psychological Association considers homosexuality to be a mental illness. Sixty-three percent of clinicians were reported to have told participants that they were not really homosexual. Nearly all participants were told that gay lives were inherently unhappy. Sixty-seven percent of therapists told their clients that therapy would make them heterosexual or bisexual (despite the lack of empirical evidence for such claims). It is notable that some clients were coerced into therapy by religious colleges or universities; others were strongly encouraged to report the story of their success in treatment to the media. For some individuals attending religious universities, confidentiality was breached without consent when therapists spoke to religious authorities about the client's same-sex attraction. Some of the participants said they pretended therapy was helping because of the pressure they felt from their therapists.

Schroeder and Shidlo (2001b) provide preliminary information on the actual experiences of individuals undergoing conversion therapies. Their study was not conducted to understand the positive or negative outcomes of such therapy, but rather to gain a better understanding of the practice itself, as told by those who experienced it. The results suggest that many—although not all—practitioners of sexual conversion therapy are practicing in a questionable manner, according to the ethical codes of most mental health organizations.

The American Psychological Association's resolution on appropriate therapeutic response to sexual orientation (American Psychological Association, 1998) does not openly oppose conversion therapies. However, the resolution states that the Association "opposes portrayals of lesbian, gay, and bisexual youth and adults as mentally ill due to their sexual orientation" (p. 934). Though it is not a professional standard that can be enforced, this statement strongly suggests that the American Psychological Association would discourage members from practicing conversion therapies. The American Psychiatric Association (1998, 2000) position paper regarding sexual conversion or reorientation therapies makes a stronger declaration against conversion therapies: "The potential risks of 'reparative therapy' are great, including depression, anxiety, and self-destructive behavior, since therapist alignment with societal prejudices against homosexuality may reinforce self-hatred" (American Psychiatric Association, 1998, as cited in Drescher, 2001, p. 203). The recommendations of the American Psychiatric Association were to affirm its 1973 position that homosexuality per se is not a diagnosable mental disorder; that psychotherapists "should not determine the goal of treatment either coercively or through subtle influence," and that the reparative therapy literature "not only ignores the impact of social stigma in motivating efforts to cure homosexuality, it is a literature that actively stigmatizes homosexuality as well . . . [and] tends to overstate the treatment's accomplishments while neglecting any potential risks to patients" (p. 206).

Both psychoanalysts and behavior therapists have a history of attempting to treat homosexuality. Behavioral therapies have tended to use aversive conditioning procedures. Clients who formerly underwent such treatment report a greater sense of harm than do clients who have undergone other forms of sexual reorientation or "reparative" therapy (Shidlo & Schroeder, 2002). Clients may suffer from increased self-hatred, sexual dysfunction, and other emotional disorders as a result of aversive conditioning to change sexual orientation (Schroeder & Shidlo, 2001a). Although such therapies may change behavior patterns, clients rarely report a change in their sexual orientation. Unfortunately, these treatments are not a thing of the past, and are still conducted by a minority of therapists that maintain the erroneous belief that heterosexuality is the only normal human sexuality.

Such treatments are fraught with social, political, and religious values. The political nature of these treatments can be traced back at least three decades. In 1974, Kohlenberg published results of treating a male who was sexually attracted to male children with *in vivo* desensitization. As a result of the treatment, the client reported decreased attraction to male children and an increased attraction to male adults. In other words, Kohlenberg successfully treated the pedophilia. However, when this article was published in the *Journal of Abnormal Psychology*, the editors solicited comments specifically questioning the success or failure of the treatment, because the client remained attracted to males. To this day, such confusion exists around this issue. When sexual reorientation therapists treat sexual behavior and clients begin to engage in heterosexual behavior, while continuing to have same-sex fantasies, the therapy is considered a success, because the client is no longer a "practicing homosexual." Opponents of conversion therapies often point out that treating clients who request treatment would only be valid if, indeed, these therapists also treated heterosexual clients who were asking to be gay. Such treatment, however, is geared to make homosexually oriented people heterosexually oriented, and not the other way around.

Therapist Bias

Bernstein (1993) acknowledged that all of us are "raised with opportunities to develop conditioned negative responses to same-gender sexual orientation" (p. 39). Some heterosexual individuals have stronger bias than others. LGB therapists are not exempt from negative bias either, and must also be aware of such bias that can be manifest in discomfort with certain client behavior. Therapists should therefore be willing to conduct an honest self-evaluation of discomfort and bias (Spencer & Hemmer, 1993).

Therapists who hold negative beliefs about LGB people can alter faulty perceptions by following the recommendations of Purcell et al. (1996): First, they should evaluate their beliefs and attitudes about LGB individuals; second, read current, affirmative literature on LGB issues; and third, have ongoing, direct experience with LGB people or clients. Biased reactions may be negatively reinforced by avoidance of LGB people. Thus, exposure is a useful technique to combat avoidance. The fourth recommendation is to develop research, training guidelines, and policies that support LGB clients. This final recommendation has been followed by the behavioral health associations discussed in this chapter that have developed guidelines.

Most therapists are well-meaning individuals who want to do the best for their clients. How, therefore, does one recognize negative bias? Certainly individuals who are hostile to LGB people can recognize this and should refer any LGB clients to LGB-affirmative therapists. However, such individuals may not even know that their clients are LGB, because they may avoid asking questions about sexual orientation out of fear of exposure to LGB people (Spencer & Hemmer, 1993). We recommend that therapists ask themselves the following questions regarding their response to LGB clients:

1. Do I believe that LGB people are immoral or disordered simply because of their sexual orientation?
2. Am I anxious when I meet a client who exhibits gender-atypical behavior (such as a man with strong feminine characteristics)?
3. Do I avoid asking clients about their sexual orientation?
4. When clients discuss dating or families, do I assume their partner is of the opposite sex?
5. Do I feel uncomfortable discussing sexual acts between two people of the same sex?
6. If I am uncomfortable with such discussion (item 5), do I make attempts to discourage clients from disclosing details of their sexual behavior?
7. Am I more likely to assume psychopathology if I know my client is LGB?
8. Do I diagnose personality disorders more frequently if my client is LGB?
9. Do I perceive LGB couples to have more problems than heterosexual couples?
10. Do I miss some of my clients' problem behaviors because I am afraid to discuss their sexual orientation, sex life, or relationship status?

This list of questions is not comprehensive. It serves as a starting point for self-evaluation. Therapists who answer "yes" to any of these questions would do well to seek consultation with an LGB-affirmative colleague prior to working with LGB clients.

Working within a Limited Community

One final issue that arises for therapists working in the LGB community, especially for those who are LGB themselves, is similar to issues faced by therapists in rural areas. The LGB community represents a small population within larger urban areas, and is even smaller in rural areas. When LGB therapists are also therapists of color, their potential social community is likely narrowed even further. Therapists who participate in community activities or political events, or who socialize at LGB-oriented establishments, face the strong possibility of seeing clients outside of the therapy setting. This situation does not always provide ethical dilemmas, but there may be times when therapists cannot avoid social contact that they may desire to avoid.

When therapists believe it is likely they will encounter clients in the community, they should clarify confidentiality policies to clients in advance. A therapist telling a client that she will not acknowledge him or her in public to protect the client's confidentiality, unless the client acknowledges her first, ensures that the client will not interpret a lack of acknowledgment as being ignored. Certainly, if there is misunderstanding, it can be addressed as a therapy issue. A client who believes people don't care about her may interpret her therapist's lack of acknowledgment at a local women's music festival to mean that the therapist doesn't care. The therapist can help the client challenge this cognition and discuss a more appropriate interpretation. However, it is usually better to avoid the misinterpretation altogether than to deal with it clinically after it has occurred. An LGB therapist who is likely to run into a client may simply say:

> "It is quite likely that we will see each other in settings outside of therapy. My priority is to help you as your therapist. Your relationship with me is confidential, so I will not acknowledge that I know you. I realize that can feel awkward, so I want you to know that it is a general policy. I want to make sure you are not placed in a position of needing to disclose that I am your therapist. You are welcome to say 'hello' to me if you see me, and I'll know by that action that you are giving me permission to acknowledge you as well."

This issue of encountering a client outside of the office is further complicated should the therapist be emotionally or sexually attracted to the client. LGB therapists are not more likely to be attracted to their clients than heterosexual therapists are to theirs, but the chance of seeing the client outside of therapy is increased in smaller communities. Sexual or exploitative relationships with clients are always unethical. Experts do not agree, however, on what constitutes an appropriate boundary between client and therapist. Whereas traditional psychoanalytic practice has forbidden any contact outside of the therapy session (Johnston & Farber, 1996, as cited in Williams, 1997), humanistic, cognitive, and behavioral therapies do not espouse a blanket prohibition. In fact, some have argued that dual relationships are occasionally necessary to enhance therapeutic efforts (e.g., Lazarus, 1994a; Zur, 2001). Nevertheless, a therapist should not disclose to a client that he or she finds the client sexually attractive or feels romantically inclined, because it is almost always unwarranted and countertherapeutic (Goodyear & Shumate, 1996).

If a therapist believes that he or she cannot maintain proper therapeutic boundaries with a client (i.e., nonsexual, nonexploitative), the client should be referred to another clinician at the earliest convenience, in accordance with relevant ethical standards. Our discussion here applies to any therapist who becomes attracted to a client, whether the parties involved are gay, straight, or bisexual. The issue at hand is that therapists in small communities may encounter current or former clients in public. It has been suggested that therapist awkwardness in a chance encounter models avoidance for clients, and that therapists often don't behave in humane ways when they encounter clients outside of the office (Hyman, 2002). Therapist effectiveness in small communities may be enhanced by familiarity (Zur & Lazarus, 2002). Nevertheless, therapists need to be aware of their own motivations when crossing a boundary with a client, and should be particularly careful if they feel sexually attracted to a client. Managing such feelings and modeling the management of complex interpersonal interactions can be a benefit to clients, who also must learn to manage the complexities of their relationships. In Table 9.1, we offer several suggestions for therapists who feel emotionally or sexually attracted to a client, yet are confident they can manage their feelings and ethically treat the client.

Some LGB therapists restrict certain activities to times or events when they are away from home. For example, some gay male therapists enjoy going out dancing or visiting a bathhouse, but will only do so if they are in a city different from that in which they have a clinical practice. This minimizes the chance of running into a client, especially a client that the therapist finds attractive. Other LGB therapists may choose not to participate in afterchurch coffee hours, or social events following meetings of LGB organizations, to minimize contact with clients. These decisions are completely up to the judgment of the therapist. Prohibi-

TABLE 9.1. Suggestions for Managing Complicated Feelings and Maintaining Ethical, Nonsexual, and Nonexploitative Contact

1. If you feel emotionally or sexually attracted to a client, tell a trusted colleague. Often, the act of keeping these feelings secret makes dealing with them more difficult. Discussing the attraction with a colleague may neutralize the feelings and can provide the support of a trusted confidante and advisor.

2. Take care that you do not dress or make yourself up to look more attractive on days when the client is scheduled for an appointment than on other days of the week. If you recognize this behavior in yourself, it suggests that you are not maintaining the professional distance necessary to treat the client. Do not do anything to make your office or yourself appear different for this particular client.

3. If you see the client in a social setting, keep the conversation short and polite. If he or she approaches you, saying "Hello, how are you?" or "Nice to see you" is usually sufficient.

4. You may need to leave or avoid some social situations that evoke or promote sexual feelings. For example, a therapist alone in a bar, having a few drinks, may be more vulnerable seeing a client that he or she finds sexually attractive. The mixture of alcohol and the sexually charged atmosphere of a bar, where people frequently cruise[a] one another, may impair judgment. The therapist would need to take care not to make connections with the client that could lead to flirting or actual contact.

5. Although self-disclosure is often used by CBT therapists as a therapeutic tool, especially in approaches such as DBT and FAP, all therapists must assess their motivation for any disclosure. All disclosures should be in the interest of the client, for the purpose of furthering the client's therapy. Therapists should be particularly cautious about disclosing details of their lives to a client to whom they are attracted, unless it is absolutely clear that such disclosure is in the client's best interest clinically. Even so, attraction or infatuation can obscure clinical judgment; therefore, seek consultation or supervision with a colleague.

6. Watch out for "permission-giving" beliefs to treat the client differently than you would treat other clients.

7. Do not schedule the client as the last appointment of the day or during times when other colleagues are not in the office building.

[a] Make contact with one another for the purpose of dating or sexual encounters.

tions against a therapist belonging to the same clubs or congregations as a client have been rejected by CBT theorists as maintaining a myth that clients are fragile in comparison to powerful therapists (Lazarus, 1994b). However, if the therapist believes that attending a certain event compromises either ethics or a client's treatment, he or she should not attend.

Therapists need to use clinical judgment about meeting clients in a brief social encounter. For some clients, such an encounter could be detrimental. The American Psychological Association (2002) ethics code has become more lenient than previous versions of the code in regard to multiple relationships with clients. Psychologists are to "refrain from entering into a multiple relationship if the multiple relationship could reasonably be expected to impair the psychologist's objectivity, competence, or effectiveness in performing his or her functions as a psychologist, or otherwise risk exploitation or harm to the person with whom the professional relationship exists" (American Psychological Association, 2002, p. 1065). Seeing a client in a public arena such as a concert or political rally, however, cannot be considered a multiple relationship. There may be times, however, when therapists belong to groups to which clients also belong. For example, if a psychologist or therapist is a member of a gay or lesbian bowling league and has a client on the same league, this would be a dual relationship. The psychologist would need to evaluate whether the relationship impairs his or her objectivity, or could lead to exploitation of the client. If it does not, the ethics code says that "multiple relationships that would not reasonably be expected to cause impairment or risk exploitation or harm are not unethical" (p. 1065). So playing on a bowling league to which a client also belongs may be ethical or unethical, depending on the context.

Before engaging in activities in which there may be contact with clients outside of therapy, therapists need to be self-reflective and assess whether such interactions are in the client's best interest, or whether they inappropriately meet the therapist's need for friendship or interaction. If it is the latter, the relationship may be unethical. Therapists need to know their clients. If a client is likely to have difficulty seeing the therapist in multiple roles (e.g., a client who has expressed sexual attraction to her therapist may seek a special relationship if they both belong to the same LGB-supportive church group), the therapist should minimize contact outside of therapy or refrain from the activity that sets up the multiple relationship. Clients who have been victims of sexual abuse, or who have suffered from inappropriate therapist boundary crossings in the past, will always be vulnerable, and therapists are wise to maintain strict boundaries with such clients.

LGB therapists can minimize uncomfortable or possibly unethical interactions by taking a few preemptive measures, such as asking for guest lists before attending events at which clients are likely to be present, or entering and exiting gymnasium showers only when it is clear that a client is not present. Therapists cannot, however, be expected to cease personal activities (e.g., church attendance or other functions) when there may be limited options for LGB-affirmative groups. If there are questions about the possibility of harming a client, therapists should consult with trusted senior colleagues on a particular situation.

Before moving on to final recommendations, we want to highlight again that there is no evidence that LGB therapists are more likely to be attracted to their clients than are heterosexual therapists. Furthermore, LGB therapists face awkward social situations with clients, similar to those therapists working in rural or other restricted communities. In many rural areas, there are only one or two churches, a local mall or shopping center, and one medical clinic or hospital. Rural therapists are likely to carry out their daily chores of shopping, taking children to school, and having medical checkups in the same places as their clients. Each therapist must evaluate his or her position on interactions with clients (Zur, 2001), using ethical codes as guiding principles and tailoring his or her interactions to the needs of the particular client. LGB therapists must do the same, even when they live in larger urban areas, because the LGB community serves as a restricted community within metropolitan centers. Note that we have limited our conversation to social contact that is brief and mostly unavoidable. We do not recommend that therapists engage in activities such as taking a client to dinner, as some do (e.g., Lazarus, 1994a), but concede that limiting oneself to seeing clients only in the office may impair certain CBT techniques, such as riding in an elevator with a phobic client, and that chance encounters with clients are usually not damaging to the client (Lazarus, 1994a).

RECOMMENDATIONS

In this chapter we have reviewed the ethical principles, standards, policy statements, and clinical guidelines from several of the larger mental health professional associations regarding LGB persons. Drawing from these sources, we recommend the following for cognitive-behavior therapists working with LGB clients.

- Therapists should familiarize themselves with the codes and policies of their particular professional association.
- The hallmark of CBT is that the treatments are empirically validated, both between subjects and in the individual case. CBT therapists should conduct only those therapies that have received appropriate support in the research literature.
- All professional codes of ethics require that therapists do no harm to their clients. Because certain therapies aimed at changing sexual orientation have not been shown to do so, and have been reported to cause harm to individuals, CBT therapists are

discouraged from practicing such treatments in the absence of data that demonstrate necessity and effectiveness. Aversive conditioning to try to change sexual orientation from homosexual to heterosexual has been particularly harmful to some individuals (Schroeder & Shidlo, 2001a; Shidlo & Schroeder, 2002), and therapists *should not engage* in such therapy.

- CBT therapists must separate personal, religious, and moral values from the work they do. Those who believe homosexuality and bisexuality are morally wrong should not endeavor to work with LGB clients. Likewise, therapists who believe that homosexuality and bisexuality are normal variants of human behavior must also be aware of stigma that can result from self-disclosure. Therefore, therapists should take care not to encourage any clients to disclose their sexual orientation, without first conducting a careful analysis of the costs and benefits for the particular individuals.

- CBT therapists must respect the diversity of life experiences that their clients bring to therapy. Not all people who express same-sex attraction or behavior will identify with an LGB community. CBT therapists must be culturally sensitive to their clients.

- CBT researchers are encouraged to include LGB individuals in their samples and to include sexual orientation in demographic information, so that greater knowledge of transfer of treatment effects with this population can be gathered.

Throughout this book, we have taken the approach that cognitive-behavioral therapists can practice with LGB clients in a sensitive and knowledgeable manner. By recognizing how personal values may interfere with one's understanding of LGB clients, and may ultimately effect a treatment plan, CBT therapists can self-monitor to provide treatment that promotes the emotional well-being of such clients.

The Past and the Future of Cognitive-Behavioral Therapy with Lesbian, Gay, and Bisexual Clients

We have maintained two equally important goals in writing this book, presenting information about LGB issues for therapists trained in CBT and the basics of CBT for those expert in LGB-affirmative therapy from other therapeutic orientations. Much of the literature on LGB psychology has been written from other than cognitive-behavioral perspectives. The behavior therapy literature has, in fact, been relatively silent on the issue (Campos & Hathaway, 1993) until very recently. Professional associations such as the Association for Advancement of Behavior Therapy, however, have, for at least the past decade, had active, special interest groups on LGB issues, and larger mental health associations (e.g., American Psychological Association) have formed committees to deal with the concerns of LGB members and clients. We have tried to provide a cognitive-behavioral conceptualization for the emotional difficulties faced by LGB clients (Cochran & Mays, 2000) and have presented examples of treatment. In doing so, we presented CBT to those who are familiar with the LGB literature but have little experience with CBT. We have also presented work with an LGB population for those cognitive-behaviorists who have little experience with this population or the LGB literature.

By virtue of growing up as members of an invisible minority, LGB individuals are subject to different stressors, in addition to the many stressors faced by their heterosexual peers. Heterosexual parents raise the majority of children who will grow up to identify as LGB. This heterosexuality is therefore the norm presented in family units, by social groups, and by the media. Given the strong rejection of same-sex attraction by much of society, recognition of one's LGB orientation can result in cognitive dissonance. The individual either denies his or her sexuality, as most do prior to coming out, or denies some aspect of the heterosexual normative environment in which he or she was raised. When one is LGB and a member of an ethnic or cultural minority group, loyalty to that group may be strained because of opposing pulls from the various groups. Religious training also can engender cognitive conflict for LGB people. An LGB person may strongly affirm his or her religious tradition and background but must then reconcile his or her sexual orientation with that tradition, which likely has a negative view of homosexuality.

CBT, thankfully, has a long history of providing frameworks for change that do not pathologize clients. The behavior analytic three-term contingency (stimulus, response, and consequence) has emphasized the impact of the environment and contingencies of reinforcement to increase behavior, adaptive and maladaptive. The addition of the cognitive "ABCs" (antecedent, belief, and consequence) accounts for beliefs that are learned and maintained. The behaviors and beliefs of an individual client, or a societal group, can be evaluated in relation to the environmental contingencies that produce and maintain them. Unfortunately, in the behavioral literature, this nonpathologizing stance toward many problems in living has not always applied to issues of sexual orientation. Throughout this book, we have presented an LGB-affirmative view. However, in reviews of some of the major texts in behavioral therapy, such a view may not be perceptible. Thus, it is useful to review where the field has been, and where it appears to be at this time, and to make recommendations for the future of CBT with LGB people.

BIAS IN THE BEHAVIORAL LITERATURE

Behavioral therapy, in particular, has been used as a means of modifying the same-sex behavior of gay men, and is therefore suspect to many LGB people. This includes LGB therapists, and therapists interested in providing affirmative psychotherapy to LGB individuals. Like classical psychoanalysis, behaviorism, until recently, held a strong bias in favor of heterosexual orientation and behavior as normal and desirable.

Methodologies to "modify homosexual behavior" per se appeared in nearly all texts on behavioral treatment from the 1950s into the 1970s.

Much of the literature regarding human sexuality has a specific bias toward heterosexuality as the norm, and as the criterion by which all sexual behaviors are assessed. It is admittedly impossible to practice value-free research or clinical work (Halleck, 1971). Every therapist or researcher thus approaches her or his work with preconceived values and judgments. Judging heterosexuality to be normal per se and homosexuality to be abnormal per se is expressing a value system, even if it represents a cultural consensus. The heterosexual bias inherent in clinical psychology has also resulted in the research on the etiology of and treatments for homosexuality, and more insidiously, in research that compares gay men and lesbians to heterosexuals, with the purpose of demonstrating the abnormality of LGB people in comparison to a heterosexual norm. For example, over the past five decades, several studies have shown scientifically that homosexuality per se is not a result of or cause of psychopathology, and that there are no reliable differences between homosexuals and heterosexuals on tests of psychopathology (Hooker, 1957; Marmor, 1980). Heterosexual bias in the field and in our culture makes this and related research seem necessary. For research to demonstrate that LGB people are "normal," it needed to include a "normal" (i.e., straight) comparison group. Western culture has dictated the norm of heterosexuality, and the behavioral health fields have unquestioningly followed this dictum.

PERSISTENT CLASSIFICATION OF SAME-SEX SEXUALITY AS A "CONDITION"

The student of behaviorism and cognitive-behaviorism can easily find in many texts from the 1970s, the 1980s, and even the 1990s, protocols for "treating" homosexuality through behavior modification. Behaviorism has regrettably maintained the classifications conditioned and reinforced by the dominant culture in the same fashion as have other schools of psychotherapy. Classic texts in the field, such as those by Bandura (1969) and Dollard and Miller (1950), contain examples of behavioral theory explaining how individuals "develop" homosexual behaviors, or of ways in which behavioral therapy can treat homosexuality. It is important to realize that the societal context in which these researchers conducted their work was different than our current context, and the exploration of treatment for homosexuality was generally considered appropriate then. However, since the late 1960s, the understanding of same-sex sexual attraction has evolved and is considered by most mental health professionals to be a normal variation of human behavior.

A more sophisticated behavioral approach to human sexual arousal has been proposed by Roche and Barnes-Holmes (2002), who suggest that earlier behavioral explanations relying on simple theories of respondent or operant conditioning are inadequate to explain the complexity of human sexual arousal. The authors propose that relational frame theory (see Chapter 8) better explains the evidence that human language impacts the emergence and maintenance of sexual arousal patterns. This intriguing article, however, unfortunately includes references to 1970s (and 1990s) research on behavior modification for same-sex sexual arousal that may be disturbing to LGB readers. Nevertheless, the emphasis on derived stimulus relations in relational frame theory is consistent with feminist and constructivist understandings of sexual orientation, although, like all behavioral theories, the former relies heavily on the experimental laboratory for empirical validation. The theory, as described, could help to explain how humans develop sexual arousal patterns for same- and opposite-sex stimuli. An LGB-affirmative approach would reject judgment on same-sex arousal patterns as deviant or fetishistic,[1] and a truly behavioral approach would make no claims for moral superiority of any one behavior over another.

In the early 1970s, mental health professional organizations and their leaders began to remove the pathological label of "homosexuality" as a diagnosis. Davison (1976)—who had been an active proponent of sexual reorientation earlier in his career—questioned the ethics of using behavioral technology to treat LGB individuals who seek therapy primarily because of the pressures society places on them to conform to a heterosexual standard. Certainly, these arguments opposing treatment of homosexuality after the removal of the diagnosis from the DSM had been heard in other quarters, but texts on behavioral therapy continued to reflect heterosexual bias nearly to the end of the 20th century.

Much of the literature published in the 1980s included disclaimers that the issue was not sexual "preference" per se, but rather other deviations of sexual attraction or behavior. However, the language found in several prominent texts showed a continued bias toward the pathology model of homosexuality. For example Adams, Tollison, and Carson, in a chapter on sexual deviations (1981), state:

> What constitutes an "appropriate" pattern of sexual arousal is currently a topic of active debate among mental health professionals, politicians, and society. Traditionally, "normal" sexuality has referred to, and been limited to, heterosexual arousal and behavior. However, the gay rights movement has recently challenged this limited conception

of normal sexual behavior and has succeeded in persuading the American Psychiatric Association to remove homosexuality from the classification of deviant sexual orientations. (p. 330)

The implication here is that pressure from the "gay rights movement" led to the decision of the American Psychiatric Association, therefore calling into question the empirical basis for the removal of homosexuality.[2] The historical account of the change in diagnosis would suggest that it was, indeed, pressure of gay and lesbian activist groups that led to the American Psychiatric Association allowing panel discussion that presented a view opposing the pathological stance (Bayer, 1981/1987) as well as greater openness to data (such as Hooker, 1957) that had formerly been explained away or discounted. Although this political pressure did result in the possibility of initiating and completing research that does not assume pathology, it was this ongoing empirical evidence, combined with the shifting societal context, that resulted in changes in diagnosis over the past several decades.

Claims that the American Psychiatric Association, the American Psychological Association, and the National Association of Social Workers have simply succumbed to political pressure do not reflect scientific data. Furthermore, the standards applied to the social and political changes toward individuals with same-sex sexual attractions are not the same standards applied to other disenfranchised groups in which psychological and political factors overlap. Social and political forces have resulted in changes in our understanding and interpretation of race differences in intelligence, questioning the validity of IQ tests developed by and normed on primarily white, European Americans for evaluating intelligence in ethnic/minority groups.

Changes in test construction and administration to make them more racially inclusive have met with very little resistance from the scientific community. However, in the case of sexual orientation, researchers and theorists continue to make judgments on same-sex attraction per se—moral grounds in the guise of science. There is no scientifically sound reason to attempt to change sexual orientation, because it has never been demonstrated that varieties of sexual orientation are not simply natural variations in human behavior. The burden of proof here should be that those who claim it is a disorder clearly demonstrate so in unbiased, scientifically sound research.

The psychotherapy literature also contains bias that is unintentional—that is, studies that do not state a preference for heterosexual behavior as the norm, yet ignore issues facing LGB men and women. Issues pertaining to same-sex couples, for example, are largely missing in the research on behavioral and cognitive-behavioral couple therapy.

There also are problems with the underrepresentation of CBT research in regard to LGB populations. For example, many people are doing research on gay and lesbian couples (cf. Kurdek 1992, 1998), but few, if any, utilize a specific cognitive or behavioral paradigm. Also, many research questionnaires and demographic inquiries that offer forced choices of "married, single, divorced" are written with the apparent assumption that participants who identify as unmarried in clinical outcome studies are in fact heterosexual and single. Writers who use such wording overlook the possibility that individuals may be gay or lesbian and partnered, but unlikely to check a box stating that they are "married" when, in fact, most states prohibit same-sex marriage. This may confound studies comparing "single" with "married" participants. Many assessment tools also use terminology that excludes sexual minorities; for example, some measures of social phobia assess "heterosocial competence" and/or "anxiety about speaking with someone attractive of the opposite sex" (e.g., the Social Avoidance and Distress Scale; Mattick & Clarke, 1998; Watson & Friend, 1969; as cited in Antony et al., 2001, pp. 417–419), whereas gay or lesbian people may have greater anxiety when talking with an attractive person of the same sex, which is similar to a heterosexual person's anxiety around the opposite sex. The Mood-Related Pleasant Events Schedule (MacPhillamy, & Lewinsohn, 1982) at least moves in the right direction by including items such as "meeting someone new of the same sex," which would, of course, mean something different for an LGB person than for a heterosexual one. The Liebowitz Social Anxiety Scale (Liebowitz, 1987; as cited in Antony et al., 2001, pp. 414–415) includes the item "trying to pick someone up," which is appropriately gender-neutral.

INVESTIGATING DIVERSITY IN CLINICAL TRIALS OF COGNITIVE-BEHAVIORAL THERAPY

Despite the emphasis among CBT scholars on empirical outcomes, application of CBT with diverse populations has not been thoroughly investigated. This may in part be due to the well-established benefit of CBT, such that utilization of the treatments with diverse populations has been assumed. The research on variables related to CBT and on LGB people has, therefore, remained distinct. Indeed, all too frequently, clinical outcome trials do not ask for information regarding sexual orientation when recruiting research participants, and it is unclear whether this population is adequately represented in clinical trials (Goldfried, 2001; Martell, 2001). Ethnic and other culturally diverse groups are also frequently underrepresented in outcome research (e.g., Guthrie, 1997).

The lack of sexual-orientation information in CBT clinical trials may in part be due to the great complexity involved in assessing sexual orientation and sexual practices. For example, not all men who have sex with men, or women who have sex with women, identify as LGB. Sexual behavior, sexual identity, and sexual orientation are unique constructs and, if treated as the same, would lead to confounds in study results. Adding the descriptors of LGB to demographic information will still neglect those individuals who do not identify as such, but who may frequently engage in same-sex sexual behavior. Likewise, those who may be in committed, long-term, same-sex relationships but do not identify with a larger LGB community might also be excluded. Despite all of these problems, although some people might go unrecognized if demographic information included sexual orientation, it would still be an improvement over current practices. The problem is not only one of excluding a particular group but also of compromising research findings. These biases must be addressed in mainstream literature (Goldfried, 2001).

It has also been suggested that researchers formulate questions in terms of sexual fantasies, arousal, and behavior, rather than in terms of an identified sexual orientation, so that samples could be classified more accurately, without using terminology that participants themselves do not use (Savin-Williams, 2001). Until that time, however, research on behavioral and CBT must be reviewed in light of research on LGB people to make the therapies culturally relevant to this population.

LGB adults who present for therapy have difficulties in life similar to those of their heterosexual counterparts. Their problems are not due to their sexual orientation (American Psychological Association, 2000), thought their problems can stem from the larger society's response to their sexual orientation. Having a sexual orientation that differs from the majority norm can exacerbate problems faced by LGB individuals. As we discussed in earlier chapters, LGB individuals may develop negative attitudes toward themselves that are reinforced by a heterocentric culture. For the many LGB individuals who arrive at adulthood without developing negative beliefs about themselves, or dysfunctional behaviors resulting from attempts at hiding their sexual orientation, there are new challenges to face.

One of the earliest tasks in late adolescence or early adulthood is "coming out," or disclosing one's sexual identity to family and friends. We discussed this process in Chapter 1. This period of disclosure can be a time of great distress, and it is likely that many therapists will see clients during this period. Each individual is different, and therapists need to conduct a good behavioral assessment (Chapter 2), but, often, depression and anxiety accompany this stage of LGB development. The subculture that has developed into LGB communities is vibrant and socially supportive for most LGB individuals. However, the predominant social venue for many LGB adults is the local bar or nightclub. Given such limited options, the potential for drug and alcohol abuse is high.

At the same time, most LGB adults are looking for similar things as are heterosexual adults: a secure home, a loving relationship, friends, and meaningful employment. All these things are attainable for LGB adults. Yet keep in mind that LGB individuals can be subject to abuse and rejection by their families, most communities do not afford protection from discrimination in work and housing for LGB individuals, and LGB relationships face societal pressures that heterosexual couples do not face. Although the lesbian community has rejected traditional patriarchal views of feminine beauty, the gay male community has incorporated idealized images of masculine youth and beauty to market everything from gay cruises to AIDS medications. Gay men often face aging with the dread of losing social status or potential for finding intimate partners because of the culture of youth that has been promulgated by the gay media.

LOOKING TO THE FUTURE

We have presented the basic premises of CBT derived from social learning theory and applied behavior analysis. Many of the empirically validated treatments (Chambless et al., 1998) for depression, anxiety disorders, and relationship distress are CBTs. However, the literature on LGB individuals rarely emphasizes CBT. We have suggested in our introduction that heterosexist bias in early CBT literature may be at the heart of this. LGB researchers have turned to developmental and social psychology to understand better the impact of stigma and prejudice. Feminist clinicians (e.g., Brown, 1994) have denounced patriarchal biases in traditional empirical psychology. The strong empirical tradition in CBT may be understood in opposition to feminist or qualitative studies. We have suggested that CBT is an expanding science. Strong allegiance to scientific verification has not stopped the field from examining a variety of approaches.

Cognitive-behavioral approaches to specific disorders have demonstrated strong empirical support. We provided examples of CBT with depression, social phobia, generalized anxiety disorders, and couple therapy. We also provided a brief overview of CBT treatment for posttraumatic stress disorder, obsessive–compulsive disorder, substance abuse, and grief and bereavement. More recently, researchers have begun to evaluate concepts that are further expanding the field of CBT. Newer behavioral methodologies have emphasized the need for clients to fully experience the joys and sufferings of living a human life. Concepts such as acceptance and mindfulness have been added to traditional methodologies that emphasize change. Behavior therapy has not given up on changing thoughts and behaviors; this is still the ultimate goal. However, many conditions in which human beings find themselves cannot be changed. Frantic attempts to rid oneself of negative thoughts and feelings can result in further suffering. So acceptance is a necessary component.

It may be the case that many LGB clinicians have remained uninterested in CBT, because they believe it to be mechanical and non-affirming of clients. This has never been the case. Few clients can be motivated to evaluate and change their thoughts and behaviors without having first developed a positive relationship with their therapists. The importance of the therapeutic relationship has been discussed in early works on clinical behavior therapy (e.g., Goldfried & Davison, 1976/1994). More recently, behavior therapists (e.g., Kohlenberg, & Tsai, 1991) have focused on the therapeutic relationship as the major arena in which behavior change occurs.

Why have CBT therapists and researchers written so little about working with LGB clients? Certainly, early bias in the field included LGB individuals only as a group of people to be treated for their sexual orientation. However, this belief no longer dominates the field. It has not been clear that LGB individuals present a unique population to be studied. We submit that there has been a tacit assumption that treatments will generalize to LGB clients, because sexual orientation is not a significant variable that would make these individuals different from standard clinical samples. In fact, many LGB individuals have more than likely been participants in treatment outcome research, but studies have not captured the relevant demographic information that would tell us unequivocally that this is true (Martell, 2001).

Researchers and therapists must look at the larger contextual factors that have an impact on clients' lives. The beauty of CBT has always been the emphasis on environmental influences on behavior and learning histories. It may not be the place of CBT therapists or associations to seek political change, but as these changes occur, clients will present with a different understanding of themselves and their problems. LGB clients who live and work in parts of the world where more conservative beliefs are commonplace have to cope with different issues than do those who live in large, liberal, urban areas.

Future research could help us understand whether outcomes of the state-of-the-art treatments we have described in this book will vary with an LGB population. Given the invalidating and often hostile environment in which LGB individuals are raised, evaluating whether many are prone to negative core beliefs about themselves also needs exploration. Likewise, understanding how the many LGB individuals who develop positive identities in the midst of adversity did so can contribute to a burgeoning understanding of resilience processes (Masten, 2001). As we stated earlier, LGB individuals are at high risk for victimization or harassment. In the face of the HIV epidemic, it is important to understand the contextual factors that play a role in sexual risk taking behavior, as well as in health maintenance behavior (e.g., Stall et al., 2002).

Cognitive-behavioral approaches will continue to be useful to individuals, couples, and groups of LGB individuals. Ultimately, however, the lives of LGB clients are improved by major contextual shifts in societal perceptions and tolerance for different sexual orientations. Insofar as LGB-affirmative religious, political, and cultural leaders continue to make inroads into legal protections and maintenance of basic civil rights for LGB people, incidences of psychological problems are likely to decrease. However, as long as cultural prejudice still allows for the kind of hatred and violence that has been leveled against LGB people, behavioral health professionals will be needed. LGB therapists have at their disposal solid treatments for the problems faced by many of their clients. CBT therapists, who have not had formal training in working with LGB individuals, have the opportunity to learn about a culturally rich and varied population. We hope this book provides a springboard for readers to seek further training and that the lives of LGB clients continue to be improved as a result.

Resources

GAY, LESBIAN, AND BISEXUAL ORGANIZATIONS

American Psychological Association
Division 44—Society for the Psychological Study of Lesbian, Gay, and
    Bisexual Issues: *www.apa.org/about/division/div44.html*
Position statements on LGB issues: *www.apa.org/pi/statemen.html*
Committee on Lesbian, Gay, and Bisexual Concerns: *www.apa.org/pi/lgbc/*
    homepage.html

Association of Gay and Lesbian Psychiatrists
4514 Chester Avenue
Philadelphia, PA 19143-3707
www.aglp.org

Human Rights Campaign Fund
www.hrc.org

National Gay and Lesbian Task Force
www.ngltf.org

ORGANIZATIONS FOR FRIENDS AND FAMILIES

AFFIRM
c/o Marvin R. Goldfried, PhD
Psychology Department
SUNY Stony Brook
Stony Brook, NY 11794-2500

Parents and Friends of Lesbians and Gays (PFLAG)
www.pflag.org

Local chapters exist throughout the country and can be located by
contacted the main address.

COGNITIVE-BEHAVIORAL THERAPY
ASSOCIATIONS AND TRAINING ORGANIZATIONS

Association for Advancement of Behavior Therapy
305 Seventh Avenue
New York, NY 10001-6008
www.aabt.org

Association of Behavior Analysis
1219 South Park Street
Kalamazoo, MI 49001
www.abainternational.org

Albert Ellis Institute
45 East 65th Street
New York, NY 10021
www.rebt.org

Beck Institute for Cognitive Therapy and Research
Suite 700, GSB Building
City Line and Belmont Aveune
Bala Cynwyd, PA 19004-1610
www.beckinstitute.org

Behavioral Technology Transfer Group
4556 University Way, NE, Suite 221
Seattle, WA 98105
www.behavioraltech.com

International Association of Cognitive Psychotherapy
http://iacp.asu.edu

Frequency and Acceptability of Partner Behavior

Andrew Christensen, PhD, and Neil S. Jacobson, PhD

Couple ID _____   Date _____

INSTRUCTIONS

In every relationship, there are positive behaviors that individuals like their partner to do, and negative behaviors that individuals don't like their partner to do. The following pages list typical behaviors that can cause relationship satisfaction or dissatisfaction. For each behavior listed below:

A) Give an estimate of the frequency of that behavior in the *past month*. Estimate the number of times (0–9) that behavior has occurred this past month either per day, week, or month. For instance, if a behavior occurred twice a week, you can either estimate it as 2 times per week or 8 times per month. In the example below, the spouse indicated that his or her partner initiated physical affection about 2 times per week in the last month. If a behavior occurred at least once in the past month, do NOT estimate it as zero times per day or zero times per week.

B) After you have estimated the frequency of the behavior in the past month, then rate how acceptable it is to you that this behavior has occurred at the specified frequency in the past month. Use the low end of the scale to rate behaviors whose frequency in the last month is unacceptable, intolerable, and unbearable. Use the high end of the scale to rate behaviors whose frequency in the last month is acceptable, even desirable. *If the behavior has not happened in the last month, respond with zero times per month, then rate how acceptable it is to you that the behavior has not happened in the past month.*

POSITIVE PARTNER BEHAVIORS

1. *In the past month*, my partner was physically affectionate (e.g., held my hand, kissed me, hugged me, put arm around me, responded when I initiated affection)

Frequency: _____ times per: Day   Week   Month   (*circle one*)

Acceptability: How acceptable is it to you that your partner was physically affectionate *at this frequency in the past month*?

Totally Unacceptable   0   1   2   3   4   5   6   7   8   9   *Totally Acceptable*

2. *In the past month*, my partner was verbally affectionate (e.g., complimented me, told me he or she loves me, said nice things)

Frequency: _____ times per: Day   Week   Month   (*circle one*)

Acceptability: How acceptable is it to you that your partner was verbally affectionate at this frequency in the past month?

Totally Unacceptable   0   1   2   3   4   5   6   7   8   9   *Totally Acceptable*

3. *In the past month*, my partner did housework (include times when partner initiated the housework as well as when you suggested it and partner did it—for example, cooked, did the dishes, cleaned the house, did the laundry, went grocery shopping, washed car, took out the trash)

Frequency: _____ times per: Day Week Month (*circle one*)

Acceptability: How acceptable is it to you that your partner did housework *at this frequency in the past month*?

Totally Unacceptable   0   1   2   3   4   5   6   7   8   9   *Totally Acceptable*

4. *In the past month*, my partner did child care (e.g., took care of the children, helped them with homework, played with them, disciplined them) [*Note*: If you and your partner do not care for children, please write N/A next to this item, leave the bubbles blank, and move on to the next item.]

Frequency: _____ times per: Day   Week   Month   (*circle one*)

Acceptability: How acceptable is it to you that your partner did childcare *at this frequency in the past month*?

Totally Unacceptable   0   1   2   3   4   5   6   7   8   9   *Totally Acceptable*

5. *In the past month*, my partner confided in me (e.g., shared with me what he or she felt, confided in me his or her successes and failures)

Frequency: _____ times per: Day Week Month (*circle one*)

Acceptability: How acceptable is it to you that your partner confided in you *at this frequency in the past month*?

Totally Unacceptable 0 1 2 3 4 5 6 7 8 9 *Totally Acceptable*

6. *In the past month*, my partner engaged in sexual activity with me (e.g., can include sexual intercourse or any other significant sexual activity, whether initiated by you or your partner)

Frequency: _____ times per: Day Week Month (*circle one*)

Acceptability: How acceptable is it to you that your partner engaged in sexual activity *at this frequency in the past month*?

Totally Unacceptable 0 1 2 3 4 5 6 7 8 9 *Totally Acceptable*

7. *In the past month*, my partner was supportive of me when I had problems (e.g., listened to my problems, sympathized with me, helped me out with my difficulties)

Frequency: _____ times per: Day Week Month (*circle one*)

Acceptability: How acceptable is it to you that your partner was supportive of you *at this frequency in the past month*?

Totally Unacceptable 0 1 2 3 4 5 6 7 8 9 *Totally Acceptable*

8. *In the past month*, my partner did social or recreational activities with me (e.g., went to movies, dinner, concerts, hiking, etc. with me, include times when partner initiated these events as well as times when you or others initiated them)

Frequency: _____ times per: Day Week Month (*circle one*)

Acceptability: How acceptable is it to you that your partner did social activities *at this frequency in the past month*?

Totally Unacceptable 0 1 2 3 4 5 6 7 8 9 *Totally Acceptable*

9. *In the past month*, my partner socialized with *my* family or *my* friends (e.g., visited my family or friends with me, was responsive when they called, joined me for outings with my family or friends)

Frequency: _____ times per: Day Week Month (*circle one*)

Acceptability: How acceptable is it to you that your partner socialized with your friends *at this frequency in the past month*?

Totally Unacceptable 0 1 2 3 4 5 6 7 8 9 *Totally Acceptable*

10. *In the past month*, my partner discussed problems in our relationship with me and tried to solve those problems (e.g., talked with me about relationship problems, tried to solve those problems constructively)

Frequency: _____ times per: Day   Week   Month   (*circle one*)

Acceptability: How acceptable is it to you that your partner discussed problems with you *at this frequency in the past month*?

Totally Unacceptable   0   1   2   3   4   5   6   7   8   9   *Totally Acceptable*

11. *In the past month*, my partner participated in the financial responsibilities of the family (e.g., helped make financial decisions, paid bills, consulted me before making major purchases)

Frequency: _____ times per: Day   Week   Month   (*circle one*)

Acceptability: How acceptable is it to you that your partner participated in finances *at this frequency in the past month*?

Totally Unacceptable   0   1   2   3   4   5   6   7   8   9   *Totally Acceptable*

12. Positive behavior(s) not included that you found important *in the last month*. Behavior: _____

Frequency: _____ times per: Day   Week   Month   (*circle one*)

Acceptability: How acceptable is it to you that your partner did this positive behavior *at this frequency in the past month*?

Totally Unacceptable   0   1   2   3   4   5   6   7   8   9   *Totally Acceptable*

NEGATIVE PARTNER BEHAVIORS

13. *In the past month*, my partner was critical of me (e.g., blamed me for problems, put down what I did, made accusations about me)

Frequency: _____ times per: Day   Week   Month   (*circle one*)

Acceptability: How acceptable is it to you that your partner was critical of you *at this frequency in the past month*?

Totally Unacceptable   0   1   2   3   4   5   6   7   8   9   *Totally Acceptable*

14. *In the past month*, my partner was dishonest with me (e.g., lied to me, failed to tell me things I wanted or needed to know, twisted the facts so I didn't find out what really happened)

Frequency: _____ times per: Day   Week   Month   (*circle one*)

Acceptability: How acceptable is it to you that your partner was dishonest with you *at this frequency in the past month*?

Totally Unacceptable   0   1   2   3   4   5   6   7   8   9   *Totally Acceptable*

15. *In the past month*, my partner was inappropriate with members of the same or opposite sex (e.g., was too flirtatious with other men/women, had secret meetings with them, made passes at them, or had affairs)

Frequency: _____ times per: Day   Week   Month   (*circle one*)

Acceptability: How acceptable is it to you that your partner was sexually inappropriate *at this frequency in the past month*?

Totally Unacceptable   0   1   2   3   4   5   6   7   8   9   *Totally Acceptable*

16. *In the past month*, my partner did not follow through with his or her agreements (e.g., didn't do what he or she said he or she would do, went back on his or her word)

Frequency: _____ times per: Day   Week   Month   (*circle one*)

Acceptability: How acceptable is it to you that your partner did not follow agreements *at this frequency in the past month*?

Totally Unacceptable   0   1   2   3   4   5   6   7   8   9   *Totally Acceptable*

17. *In the past month*, my partner was verbally abusive with me (e.g., swore at me, called me names, yelled or screamed)

Frequency: _____ times per: Day   Week   Month   (*circle one*)

Acceptability: How acceptable is it to you that your partner was verbally abusive *at this frequency in the past month*?

Totally Unacceptable   0   1   2   3   4   5   6   7   8   9   *Totally Acceptable*

18. *In the past month*, my partner was physically abusive with me (e.g., pushed, shoved, kicked, bit or hit me, or threw things)

Frequency: _____ times per: Day   Week   Month   (*circle one*)

Acceptability: How acceptable is it to you that your partner was physically abusive *at this frequency in the past month*?

Totally Unacceptable   0   1   2   3   4   5   6   7   8   9   *Totally Acceptable*

19. *In the past month*, my partner was controlling and bossy (e.g., did things without consulting with me first, insisted on his or her way, didn't listen to what I wanted, manipulated things so he or she got what he or she wanted)

Frequency: _____ times per: Day   Week   Month   (*circle one*)

Acceptability: How acceptable is it to you that your partner was controlling and bossy *at this frequency in the past month*?

Totally Unacceptable   0   1   2   3   4   5   6   7   8   9   *Totally Acceptable*

20. *In the past month*, my partner invaded my privacy (e.g., opened my mail, listened in on my conversations with friends or family)

Frequency: _____ times per: Day   Week   Month   (*circle one*)

Acceptability: How acceptable is it to you that your partner invaded your privacy *at this frequency in the past month*?

Totally Unacceptable   0   1   2   3   4   5   6   7   8   9   *Totally Acceptable*

21. *In the past month*, my partner engaged in addictive behavior (such as smoking, using drugs, drinking alcohol, etc.) that bothered me. *Note*: Please include what the behavior was _____.

Frequency: _____ times per: Day   Week   Month   (*circle one*)

Acceptability: How acceptable is it to you that your partner engaged in this addiction *at this frequency in the past month*?

Totally Unacceptable   0   1   2   3   4   5   6   7   8   9   *Totally Acceptable*

22. Negative behavior(s) not included that you found important *in the last month*. Behavior: _____

Frequency: _____ times per: Day   Week   Month   (*circle one*)

Acceptability: How acceptable is it to you that your partner did this negative behavior *at this frequency in the past month*?

Totally Unacceptable   0   1   2   3   4   5   6   7   8   9   *Totally Acceptable*

ITEMS OF MOST CONCERN TO YOU

Out of the behaviors you rated on this questionnaire, what are the 5 behaviors (positive or negative) that were of most concern to you or that troubled you the most *in the last month*? For example, if item 13 was of most concern, you would write the number 13, then indicate the issue was criticism (see example below). PLEASE DO NOT put more than one item on each line, and please do your best to choose 5 items as requested.

EXAMPLE:

Item of Most Concern: Item # on this questionnaire _13___
Item Topic ____*critical of me*_____

WHAT IS *YOUR*:

Item of Most Concern: Item # on this questionnaire _____
Item Topic _____

Item of 2nd Most Concern: Item # on this questionnaire _____
Item Topic _____

Item of 3rd Most Concern: Item # on this questionnaire _____
Item Topic _____

Item of 4th Most Concern: Item # on this questionnaire _____
Item Topic _____

Item of 5th Most Concern: Item # on this questionnaire _____
Item Topic _____

IBCT Feedback Session Summary Sheet

In helping couples to address problems in their relationship, therapists try to answer several questions. The following is a summary sheet of information presented to you in your feedback session:

What are the *themes* that are problematic for this couple?

_____

_____

_____

What factors about each partner make him or her *vulnerable* to these themes?

Partner 1 _____

_____

_____

Partner 2 _____

_____

_____

How has this couple become divided or *polarized*?

_____

_____

_____

How can therapy help?

_____

_____

_____

Notes

PREFACE

1. We are not addressing the issues of people who consider themselves transgendered or intergendered in this book because the data are only recently being
   collected on this population. Furthermore, it is generally understood that issues
   of gender identity are separate from those of sexual orientation or identity. Both
   transgendered and intergendered people may be considered broadly as part of a
   sexual minority that includes LGB people, but the complex area of gender is beyond the scope of this book. "Transgender" broadly means those who do not follow traditional gender classifications, whereas "transsexual" specifically means
   those individuals that are phenotypically different from their understanding of
   themselves as either male or female. "Intergender" refers to individuals who are
   born with genitalia of both sexes.

CHAPTER ONE

1. The AIDS pandemic brought the gay and lesbian communities together to form
   organizations such as Gay Men's Health Crisis (GMHC) in New York City to
   deal with a situation perceived as being largely ignored by the Reagan administration. However, it also saw a resurgence of anti-gay rhetoric as televangelists
   decried AIDS as a sign of "God's wrath" against homosexuality. It is a curious argument given that lesbians are in a demographic group with least risk for HIV/
   AIDS.
2. Kinsey, Pomeroy, and Martin (1948) developed a well-known scale of sexual
   identity, often referred to as the "Kinsey Scale." Individuals scoring 0 on this
   scale would consider themselves to be exclusively heterosexual, whereas a
   "Kinsey 6" would identify them as exclusively homosexual.
3. The Cochran et al. (2003) study differed from and improved on earlier studies

that used sexual behavior to determine sexual orientation. They used data from individuals that self-identified as LGB or heterosexual, thus reducing the possibility of misclassification bias.

4. Although the term "queer" has been used by some LGB groups as a general identifier, such as the group "Queer Nation," the term historically has been a pejorative label and is considered offensive by some.

CHAPTER TWO

1. Note that the idea of "ABC" proposed by Ellis and other cognitive therapists is different from the ABC of the three-point contingency used in behavior analysis. For the cognitive therapist, the crux of the analysis is the belief, and the activation of a belief leading to a particular consequence. For the behavior analyst, all behavior (public or private) is contextually based, and each point of the contingency, the antecedent to a behavior (e.g., seeing an old friend on the street), the behavior itself (e.g., offering one's hand in greeting), and the consequence (e.g., having a brief, pleasant conversation about old times) are equally important in maintaining behavior.

2. In Beck's model of cognitive therapy, dormant negative core beliefs or schemas may be reactivated when the pressure of the environment increases.

CHAPTER THREE

1. Assertiveness training provides a good example of the crossover between working between skills acquisition and emotion management, because lack of assertiveness is frequently consequent to both limited behavioral skills repertoires and inhibitions due to fear and social anxiety.

2. The therapist needs to keep in mind that certain disorders such as attention-deficit/hyperactivity disorder, generalized anxiety disorder, and depression can be exacerbated by substance use. This is also true for relationship difficulties, which are frequently worsened when couples use mind-altering substances. All of these factors need to be taken into account when the therapist collaborates with the client about his or her choices regarding substance use. Clients may also be misusing prescription medications, and therapists are wise to assess for this with clients who are also under the care of a physician.

3. Clients should be asked to arrive several minutes prior to the beginning of their session to complete the forms. This way, time is not taken during the actual session. Forms can be kept in a convenient location in the waiting area, with pens or pencils available.

4. One of the earliest cognitive schools of therapy was rational–emotive therapy (Ellis, 1962), which is now referred to as rational–emotive behavior therapy, or REBT. Closely related to REBT is Beck's (1976) cognitive therapy. Both Ellis and Beck were originally trained as psychoanalysts. The theory and technique that they developed follows the empirical tradition of behavior therapy but empha-

sizes the idea that it is important to change underlying beliefs to guarantee lasting behavioral change or emotional control. The third cognitive school of thought is constructivism (Neimeyer & Mahoney, 1995). Cognitive constructivism follows the theory that knowledge does not exist in itself but is a relationship between the knower and the known. It is, therefore, an active construction of the subject's experience and action. In this model, truth is seen not as absolute but contextual (Neimeyer, 1995). The model therefore rejects the notion that there is an objective, external, reality to which an individual's beliefs are compared and rendered rational or irrational, depending on correspondence. Behavior therapy and CBT, like other forms of psychotherapy, continue to evolve. The models presented here, however, are not exclusive of each other, and many CBT theorists value ideas from all of these schools of thought. Recent ideas that are changing the face of behavior therapy are discussed in Chapter 8.

5. This is often referred to as "behavioral homework," but it is useful to think of a word that does not hold some of the negative connotations from school days. The therapist can ask the client to think of a word that is acceptable. For simplicity sake, we follow tradition and use the term "homework."

CHAPTER FOUR

1. Many excellent books on cognitive therapies provide examples of useful questions (e.g., J. S. Beck, 1995; Greenberger & Padesky, 1995).

CHAPTER SIX

1. For excellent treatments of issues faced by LGB people of color, and of the problems of ethnic and cultural bias in research, readers are directed to Fukuyama and Ferguson (2000), Greene (1994), Guthrie (1997), and Longres (1996).

2. These include biological parenting by a lesbian partner with a known or unknown sperm donor; adoption by lesbian or gay partners; surrogate pregnancy by a female friend for a gay male couple; adoption by a gay man or lesbian of his or her partner's child(ren) from a previous marriage; foster parenting; and gay men and lesbians coparenting a child conceived in any of the above ways.

CHAPTER SEVEN

1. The Subjective Units of Discomfort Scale asks clients to describe an activity or situation in which they would experience fear. A situation that elicited little to no fear would be ranked 0, whereas a situation that the client believed would elicit the most fear they have ever experienced would be rated 100. Clinicians should help clients to identify a continuum of anxiety-producing events in 5- or 10-unit increments along the scale.

CHAPTER EIGHT

1. We would like to thank Steven Hayes, Robert Kohlenberg, Kevin Kuehlwein, and Amy Wagner for reviewing portions of an early draft of this chapter, and for making important suggestions and clarifications.
2. For an exceptionally clear and understandable presentation of relational frame theory, see Blackledge (2002).
3. Engaging in unprotected anal intercourse.

CHAPTER NINE

1. The "Pink Pages" is a name for telephone directories in certain cities aimed at LGB and transgendered clientele.
2. Cognitive and behavioral therapists would learn more about appropriate therapeutic responses to sexual orientation if LGB individuals were included and tracked in mainstream CBT research (Martell, 2001). Without adequate mainstream research, LGB people remain marginalized, studied only by researchers attempting to understand LGB-positive approaches or those who continue to search for the means to "cure" LGB adults. In either case, the research develops outside of mainstream CBT research. Political and religious views confuse the issue. We have presented literature from those who promote LGB-affirmative therapies, and this book will no doubt add to that literature.

CHAPTER TEN

1. Nowhere in the article is it implied that the authors, Roche and Barnes-Holmes, hold the view that same-sex arousal is "deviant." In fact, they state that "humans are capable of responding sexually to an almost infinite variety of stimuli" (p. 151). It is unfortunate, however, that the heterosexist bias of earlier behavioral literature continues to cast a shadow on emerging theory and research.
2. Political and social pressure after events such as the famous Tuskegee study—in which researchers in Alabama (funded by the Centers for Disease Control and Prevention) had for decades deceived a sample of African American men with syphilis to stay in a study that did not allow them to receive available and effective treatment for their serious, progressive illness—forced needed changes in ethical human research guidelines. This is an example of political pressure affecting science in ways that most people recognize as wise and humane. We suggest that political influence on the way that the behavioral sciences more scientifically examine and deal with LGB issues is no less wise and humane.

References

Abramowitz, J. S., & Kalsy, S. A. (2001). Recent developments in the cognitive-behavioral treatment of obsessive–compulsive disorder. *The Behavior Analyst Today*, 2, 141–145. Retrieved January 31, 2003, from *http://www.behavior-analyst-online.org.*

Adams, H. E., Tollison, C. D., & Carson, T. P. (1981). Behavior therapy with sexual deviations. In S. M. Turner, K. S. Calhoun, & H. E. Adams (Eds.), *Handbook of clinical behavior therapy* (pp. 318–346). New York: Wiley.

Addis, M. E., Hatgis, C., Soysa, C. K., Zaslavsky, I., & Bourne, L. S. (1999). The dialectics of manual-based treatment. *the Behavior Therapist*, 22, 130–132.

Addis, M. E., & Jacobson, N. S. (1996). Reasons for depression and outcome of cognitive-behavioral psychotherapies. *Journal of Consulting and Clinical Psychology*, 64, 1417–1424.

Alberti, R. E., & Emmons, M. L. (2001). *Your perfect right* (8th ed.). San Luis Obispo, CA: Impact.

American Psychiatric Association. (1994). *Diagnostic and statistical manual of mental disorders* (4th ed.). Washington, DC: Author.

American Psychiatric Association. (1998, December). *APA position statement on psychiatric treatment and sexual orientation*. Washington, DC: Author.

American Psychiatric Association. (2000). *American Psychiatric Association Commission on Psychotherapy by Psychiatrists position statement on therapies focused on attempts to change sexual orientation (reparative or conversion therapies)*. Washington, DC: Author.

American Psychological Association. (1998). Resolution on appropriate therapeutic response to sexual orientation. Proceedings of the American Psychological Association, Incorporated, for the Legislative Year 1997. *American Psychologist*, 53, 934–935.

American Psychological Association. (2000). *Guidelines for psychotherapy with lesbian, gay and bisexual clients*. Washington, DC: Author.

American Psychological Association. (2001). *Publication manual of the American Psychological Association* (5th ed.). Washington, DC: Author.

American Psychological Association. (2002). Ethical principles of psychologists and code of conduct. *American Psychologist, 57*, 1060–1073.

Anhalt, K., Morris, T. L., Scottie, J. R., & Cohen, S. H. (2003). Student perspectives on training in gay, lesbian, and bisexual issues: A survey of behavioral clinical psychology programs. *Cognitive and Behavioral Practice, 10*(3), 255–263.

Antony, M. M., Orsillo, S. M., & Roemer, L. (2001). *Practitioner's guide to empirically based measures of anxiety.* New York: Kluwer Academic/Plenum.

Atkins, D. C. (2002). *Infidelity in marital therapy: Initial findings from a randomized clinical trial.* Unpublished doctoral dissertation, University of Washington, Seattle.

Bailey, J. M., & Pillard, R. C. (1991). A genetic study of male sexual orientation. *Archives of General Psychiatry, 48*, 1089–1096.

Bailey, J. M., Pillard, R. C., Neale, M. C., & Agyei, Y. (1993). Heritable factors influence female sexual orientation. *Archives of General Psychiatry, 50*, 217–223.

Bailey, J. M., & Zucker, K. J. (1995). Childhood sex-typed behavior and sexual orientation: A conceptual analysis and quantitative review. *Developmental Psychology, 31*, 43–55.

Bandura, A. (1969). *Principles of behavior modification.* New York: Holt, Rinehart & Winston.

Barlow, D. H. (1988). *Anxiety and its disorders: The nature and treatment of anxiety and panic* (1st ed.). New York: Guilford Press.

Barlow, D. H. (2001a). *Anxiety and its disorders: The nature and treatment of anxiety and panic* (2nd ed.). New York: Guilford Press.

Barlow, D. H. (Ed.). (2001b). *Clinical handbook of psychological disorders* (3rd ed.). New York: Guilford Press.

Barón, A., & Cramer, D. W. (2001). Potential counseling concerns of aging lesbian, gay, and bisexual clients. In R. M. Perez, K. A. DeBord, & K. J. Bieschke (Eds.), *Handbook of counseling and psychotherapy with lesbian, gay, and bisexual client* (pp. 207–223). Washington, DC: American Psychological Association.

Basseches, M. (1984). *Dialectical thinking and adult development.* Norwood, NJ: Ablex.

Baucom, D. H., & Epstein, N. (1990). *Cognitive-behavioral marital therapy.* New York: Brunner/Mazel.

Baucom, D. H., Shoham, V., Meuser, K. T., Daiuto, A. D., & Stickle, T. R. (1998). Empirically supported couple and family interventions for marital distress and adult mental health problems. *Journal of Consulting and Clinical Psychology, 66*, 53–88.

Bayer, R. (1987). *Homosexuality and American psychiatry: The politics of diagnosis.* Princeton, NJ: Princeton University Press. (Original work published 1981)

Beck, A. T. (1976). *Cognitive therapy and the emotional disorders.* New York: International Universities Press.

Beck, A. T. (1978). *Beck Hopelessness Scale.* San Antonio: Psychological Corp., Harcourt Brace & Co.

Beck, A. T. (1988). *Love is never enough.* New York: Harper & Row.

Beck, A. T., Epstein, N., Brown, G., & Steer, R. A. (1988). An inventory for measuring clinical anxiety: Psychometric properties. *Journal of Consulting and Clinical Psychology, 49*, 448–454.

Beck, A. T., Rush, A. J., Shaw, B. F., & Emery, G. (1979). *Cognitive therapy of depression*. New York: Guilford Press.

Beck, A. T., & Steer, R. A. (1988). *Manual for the Beck Hopelessness Scale*. San Antonio TX: Psychological Corp.

Beck, A. T., Steer, R. A., & Brown, G. K. (1996). *Manual for the BDI-II*. San Antonio, TX: Psychological Corp.

Beck, A. T., Ward, C. H., Mendelson, M., Mock, J., & Erbaugh, J. (1961). An inventory for measuring depression. *Archives of General Psychiatry, 4*, 561–571.

Beck, J. S. (1995). *Cognitive therapy: Basics and beyond*. New York: Guilford Press.

Bell, A. P., & Weinberg, M. S. (1978). *Homosexualities: A study of diversity among men and women*. New York: Simon & Schuster.

Bem, D. J. (1970). *Beliefs, attitudes, and human affairs*. Belmont, CA: Wadsworth.

Berman, A. L., & Jobes, D. A. (1992). Suicidal behavior of adolescents. In B. Bonger (Ed.), *Suicide: Guidelines for assessment, management and treatment* (pp. 84–105). New York: Oxford University Press.

Bernstein, G. S. (1993). Assessment and goal selection with lesbian and gay clients. *the Behavior Therapist, 16*(2), 37–40.

Blackledge, J. T. (2002). An introduction to relational frame theory: Basics and applications. *The Behavior Analyst Today, 3*, 421–433. Retrieved January 31, 2003, from *http://www.behavior-analyst-online.org*.

Blankstein, K. R., & Segal, Z. V. (2001). Cognitive assessment: Issues and methods. In K. S. Dobson (Ed.), *Handbook of cognitive-behavioral therapies* (2nd ed., pp. 40–85). New York: Guilford Press.

Blasband, D., & Peplau, L. A. (1985). Sexual exclusivity versus openness in gay couples. *Archives of Sexual Behavior, 14*, 395–412.

Blumstein, P., & Schwartz, P. (1983). *American couples: Money, work and sex*. New York: Morrow.

Boswell, J. (1980). *Christianity, social tolerance and homosexuality: Gay people in Western Europe from the beginning of the Christian era to the fourteenth century*. Chicago: University of Chicago Press.

Bradford, J., Ryan, C., & Rothblum, E. D. (1994). National Lesbian Health Care Survey: Implications for mental health care. *Journal of Consulting and Clinical Psychology, 62*, 228–242.

Brown, E. J., Turovsky, J., Heimberg, R. G., Juster, H. R., Brown, T. A., & Barlow, D. H. (1997). Validation of the Social Interaction Anxiety Scale and the Social Phobia Scale across the anxiety disorders. *Psychological Assessment, 9*, 21–27.

Brown, L. S. (1994). *Subversive dialogues: Theory in feminist therapy*. New York: Basic Books.

Brown, L. S. (1995). Lesbian identities: Concepts and issues. In A. R. D'Augelli & C. J. Patterson (Eds.), *Lesbian, gay, and bisexual identities over the lifespan: Psychological perspectives* (pp. 3–23). New York: Oxford University Press.

Burns, D. (1999). *Feeling good: The new mood therapy* (rev. ed.). New York: Wholecare. (Original work published 1980)

Bux, D. A. (1996). The epidemiology of problem drinking in gay men and lesbians: A critical review. *Clinical Psychology Review, 16*, 277–298.

Campos, P. E., & Hathaway, B. E. (1993). Behavioral research on gay issues 20 years after Davison's ethical challenge. *the Behavior Therapist, 16*, 193–197.

Carrington, C. (1999). *No place like home: Relationships and family life among lesbians and gay men*. Chicago: University of Chicago Press.

Chambless, D. L., Baker, M. J., Baucom, D. H., Beutler, L. E., Calhoun, K. S., Crits-Christoph, P., Baker, M., Johnson, B., Wood, S. R., Sue, S., Beutler, L., Williams, D. A., & McCurry, S. (1998). Update on empirically validated therapies II. *The Clinical Psychologist, 51*, 3–16.

Chan, C. S. (1995). Issues of sexual identity in an ethnic minority: The case of Chinese American lesbians, gay men, and bisexual people. In A. R. D'Augelli & C. J. Patterson, (Eds.), *Lesbian, gay, and bisexual identities over the lifespan: Psychological perspectives* (pp. 87–101). New York: Oxford University Press.

Chapman, A. L., & Dehle, C. (2002). Bridging theory and practice: A comparative analysis of integrative behavioral couple therapy and cognitive behavioral couple therapy. *Cognitive and Behavioral Practice, 9*, 150–163.

Christensen, A. (1987). Detection of conflict patterns in couples. In K. Hahlweg & M. J. Goldstein (Eds.), *Understanding major mental disorder: The contribution of family interaction research* (pp. 250–265). New York: Family Process Press.

Christensen, A., & Heavey, C. L. (1990). Gender and social structure in the demand/withdraw pattern of marital conflict. *Journal of Personality and Social Psychology, 59*, 73–81.

Christensen, A., & Heavey, C. L. (1999). Interventions for couples. *Annual Review of Psychology, 50*, 165–190.

Christensen, A., & Jacobson, N. S. (1997). *Frequency and Acceptability of Partner Behavior*. Unpublished questionnaire. (Available from Andrew Christensen, University of California, Department of Psychology, Los Angeles, CA 90095)

Christensen, A., & Jacobson, N. S. (2000). *Reconcilable differences*. New York: Guilford Press.

Christensen, A., Jacobson, N. S., & Babcock, J. C. (1995). Integrative behavioral couple therapy. In N. S. Jacobson & A. S. Gurman (Eds.), *Clinical handbook of couple therapy* (pp. 31–64). New York: Guilford Press.

Clunis, D. M., & Green, G. D. (2000). *Lesbian couples: A guide to creating healthy relationships*. Seattle: Seal Press.

Cochran, B. N., Stewart, A. J., Ginzler, J. A., & Cauce, A. M. (2002). Challenges faced by homeless sexual minorities: Comparison of gay, lesbian, bisexual, and transgender homeless adolescents with their heterosexual counterparts. *American Journal of Public Health, 92*, 773–777.

Cochran, S. D., & Mays, V. M. (2000). Relation between psychiatric syndromes and behaviorally defined sexual orientation in a sample of the US population. *American Journal of Epidemiology, 151*, 516–523.

Cochran, S. D., Sullivan, J. G., & Mays, V. M. (2003). Prevalence of mental disorders, psychological distress, and mental health services use among lesbian, gay, and bisexual adults in the United States. *Journal of Consulting and Clinical Psychology, 71*, 53–61.

Cogan, J. C. (1999). Lesbians walk the tightrope of beauty: Thin is in but femme is out. *Journal of Lesbian Studies, 3*, 77–89.

Cohen, S., & Wills, T. A. (1985). Stress, social support, and the buffering hypothesis. *Psychological Bulletin, 98*, 310–357.

Cordova, J. V. (2002). Behavior analysis and the scientific study of couples. *The

Behavior Analyst Today, *3*, 412–420. Retrieved January 31, 2003, from *http://www. behavior-analyst-online.org*.

Cordova, J. V., Jacobson, N. S., & Christensen, A. (1998). Acceptance versus change interventions in behavioral couples therapy: Impact on couples' in-session communication. *Journal of Marriage and Family Counseling*, *24*, 437–455.

Cowan, C. P., Cowan, P. A., Coie, L., & Coie, J. D. (1978). Becoming a family: The impact of a first child's birth on the couple's relationship. In W. B. Miller & L. F. Newman (Eds.), *The first child and family formation*. Chapel Hill, NC: Carolina Population Center.

Craske, M. G., Barlow, D. H., & Meadows, E. A. (2000). *Mastery of your anxiety and panic: Therapist guide for anxiety, panic, and agoraphobia* (3rd ed.). San Antonio, TX: Graywind/Psychological Corp.

Dattilio, F. M., & Padesky, C. A. (1990). *Cognitive therapy with couples*. Sarasota, FL: Professional Resource Exchange.

D'Augelli, A. R. (1998). Developmental implications of victimization of lesbian, gay, and bisexual youths. In G. M. Herek (Ed.), *Stigma and sexual orientation: Understanding prejudice against lesbians, gay men, and bisexuals* (pp. 187–210). Thousand Oaks, CA: Sage.

Davison, G. C. (1976). Homosexuality: The ethical challenge. *Journal of Consulting and Clinical Psychology*, *44*, 157–162.

Dimeff, L., Rizvi, S. L., Brown, M., & Linehan, M. M. (2000). Dialectical behavior therapy for substance abuse: A pilot application to methamphetamine-dependent women with borderline personality disorder. *Cognitive and Behavioral Practice*, *7*(4), 457–467.

DiNardo, P. A., Brown, T. A., & Barlow, D. H. (1994). Anxiety disorders interview schedule for DSM-IV: Lifetime version. San Antonio, TX: Psychological Corp.

DiPlacido, J. (1998). Minority stress among lesbians, gay men, and bisexuals: A consequence of heterosexism, homophobia, and stigmatization. In G. M. Herek (Ed.), *Stigma and sexual orientation: Understanding prejudice against lesbians, gay men, and bisexuals* (pp. 138–159). Thousand Oaks, CA: Sage.

Dollard, J., & Miller, N. E. (1950). *Personality and psychotherapy*. New York: McGraw-Hill.

Doss, B. A., & Christensen, A. (1999). *Marital couples' reports of partner behavior: Gender differences in frequency and acceptability*. Paper presented at the 33rd annual convention of the Association for Advancement of Behavior Therapy, Toronto, Ontario, Canada.

Drescher, J. (2001). Ethical concerns raised when patients seek to change same-sex attraction. *Journal of Gay and Lesbian Psychotherapy*, *5*, 181–210.

Dworkin, S. H. (1997). Female, lesbian, and Jewish: Complex and invisible. In B. Greene (Ed.), *Ethnic and cultural diversity among lesbians and gay Men* (pp. 63–87). Newbury Park, CA: Sage.

D'Zurilla, T. J., & Nezu, A. (1982). Social problem solving in adults. In P. Kendall (Ed.), *Advances in cognitive-behavioral research and therapy* (Vol. 1, pp. 201–274). New York: Academic Press.

Eidelson, R. J., & Epstein, N. (1982). Cognition and relationship maladjustment: Development of a measure of dysfunctional relationship beliefs. *Journal of Consulting and Clinical Psychology*, *50*, 715–720.

Ellis, A. (1962). *Reason and emotion in psychotherapy*. New York: Lyle Stuart.

Ellis, A. (1973). *Humanistic psychotherapy*. New York: McGraw-Hill.

Ellis, A., & Harper, R. A. (1997). *A guide to rational living* (3rd rev. ed.). North Hollywood, CA: Melvin Powers.

Ellis, L., & Ames, M. A. (1987). Neurohormonal functioning and sexual orientation: A theory of homosexuality–heterosexuality. *Psychological Bulletin, 101*, 233–255.

Eng, W., Coles, M. E., Heimberg, R. G., & Safren, S. A. (2001). Quality of life following cognitive-behavioral treatment for social anxiety disorder: Preliminary findings. *Depression and Anxiety, 13*, 192–193.

Fassinger, R. E., & Miller, B. A. (1996). Validation of an inclusive model of homosexual identity formation on a sample of gay men. *Journal of Homosexuality, 32*, 53–78.

Ferster, C. B. (1973). A functional analysis of depression. *American Psychologist, 28*, 857–870.

First, M., Spitzer, R. L., Gibbon, M., & Williams, J. B. W. (1997). User's guide for the *Structured Clinical Interview for DSM-IV Axis I Disorders: Clinical Version*. Washington DC: American Psychiatric Press.

Foa, E. B., & Goldstein, A. (1978). Continuous exposure and strict response prevention in the treatment of obsessive–compulsive neurosis. *Behavior Therapy, 9*, 821–829.

Foa, E. B., & Kozak, M. J. (1986). Emotional processing of fear: Exposure to corrective information. *Psychological Bulletin, 99*, 20–35.

Foa, E. B., & Rothbaum, B. O. (1998). *Treating the trauma of rape: Cognitive-behavioral therapy for PTSD*. New York: Guilford Press.

Foa, E. B., Rothbaum, B. O., Riggs, D. S., & Murdock, T. B. (1991). Treatment of posttraumatic stress disorder in rape victims: A comparison between cognitive-behavioral procedures and counseling. *Journal of Consulting and Clinical Psychology, 59*, 715–723.

Foa, E. B., Steketee, G., & Rothbaum, B. (1989). Behavioral/cognitive conceptualizations of posttraumatic stress disorder. *Behavior Therapy, 20*, 155–176.

Foa, E. B., Zoellner, L. A., Feeny, N. C., Hembree, E. A., & Alvarez-Conrad, J. (2002). Does imaginal exposure exacerbate PTSD symptoms? *Journal of Consulting and Clinical Psychology, 70*, 1022–1028.

Fruzzetti, A. E., & Levensky, E. R. (2000). Dialectical behavior therapy for domestic violence: Rationale and procedures. *Cognitive and Behavioral Practice, 7*(4), 435–446.

Fudge, R. C. (1996). The use of behavior therapy in the development of ethnic consciousness: A treatment model. *Cognitive and Behavioral Practice, 3*, 317–335.

Fukuyama, M. A., & Ferguson, A. D. (2000). Lesbian, gay, and bisexual people of color: Understanding cultural complexity and managing multiple oppressions. In R. M. Perez, K. A. DeBord, & K. J. Bieschke (Eds.), *Handbook of counseling and psychotherapy with lesbian, gay, and bisexual clients* (pp. 81–106). Washington, DC: American Psychological Association.

Garnets, L., Hancock, K. A., Cochran, S. D., Goodchilds, J., & Peplau, L. A. (1991). Issues in psychotherapy with lesbians and gay men: A survey of psychologists. *American Psychologist, 46*, 964–972.

Garnets, L. D. (2002). Sexual orientations in perspective. *Cultural Diversity and Ethnic Minority Psychology, 8,* 115–129.

Gilman, S. E., Cochran, S. D., Mays, V. M., Hughes, M., Ostrow, D., & Kessler, R. C. (2001). Risk of psychiatric disorders among individuals reporting same-sex sexual partners in the National Comorbidity Survey. *American Journal of Public Health, 91,* 933–939.

Gluhoski, V. (1996). Psychotherapy with dying AIDS patients and their significant others. In I. Crawford & B. Fishman (Eds.), *Psychosocial interventions in HIV disease: A stage-focused and culture-specific approach* (pp. 64–93). Northvale, NJ: Jason Aronson.

Goldfried, M. R. (2001). Integrating gay, lesbian, and bisexual issues into mainstream psychology. *American Psychologist, 56,* 977–988.

Goldfried, M. R., & Davison, G. C. (1994). *Clinical behavior therapy* (exp. ed.). New York: Wiley. (Original work published 1976)

Gollwitzer, P. M. (1999). Implementation intentions: Strong effects of simple plans. *American Psychologist, 54,* 493–503.

Gonsiorek, J. C. (1982). The use of diagnostic concepts in working with gay and lesbian populations. In J. C. Gonsiorek (Ed.), *Homosexuality and psychotherapy: A practitioner's handbook of affirmative models* (pp. 9–20). New York: Haworth Press.

Gonsiorek, J. C. (1996). Mental health and sexual orientation. In R. C. Savin-Williams & K. M. Cohen (Eds.), *The lives of lesbians, gays, and bisexuals: Children to adults* (pp. 462–478). New York: Harcourt Brace.

Gonsiorek, J. C., & Rudolph, J. (1991). Homosexual identity: Coming out and other developmental events. In J. Gonsiorek & J. Weingrich (Eds.), *Homosexuality: Research implications for public policy* (pp. 161–176). Newbury Park, CA: Sage.

Goodman, W. K., Price, L. H., Rasmussen, S. A., Mazure, C., Fleischmann, R. L., Hill, C. L., Henenger, G. R., & Charney, D. S. (1989). The Yale–Brown Obsessive–Compulsive Scale: I. Development, use, and reliability. *Archives of General Psychiatry, 46,* 1006–1011.

Goodyear, R. K., & Shumate, J. L. (1996). Perceived effects of therapist self-disclosure of attraction to clients. *Professional Psychology: Research and Practice, 27,* 613–616.

Green, R. J., Bettinger, M., & Zachs, E. (1996). Are lesbian couples fused and gay male couples disengaged? In J. Laird & R. Green (Eds.), *Lesbians and gays in couples and families* (pp. 185–230). San Francisco: Jossey-Bass.

Green, R. J., & Mitchell, V. (2002). Gay and lesbian couples in therapy: Homophobia, relational ambiguity, and social support. In A. S. Gurman & N. S. Jacobson (Eds.), *Clinical handbook of couple therapy* (3rd ed., pp. 546–568). New York: Guilford Press.

Greenan, D. E., & Tunnell, G. (2003). *Couple therapy with gay men.* New York: Guilford Press.

Greenberger, D., & Padesky, C. (1995). *Mind over mood: Changing the way you feel by changing the way you think.* New York: Guilford Press.

Greene, B. (1994). Lesbian women of color: Triple jeopardy. In L. Comas-Díaz & B. Greene (Eds.), *Women of color: Integrating ethnic and gender identities in psychotherapy* (pp. 389–427). New York: Guilford Press.

Guthrie, R. V. (1997). *Even the rat was white: A historical view of psychology* (2nd ed.). Boston: Allyn & Bacon.

Haldeman, D. C. (1994). The practice of sexual orientation conversion therapy. *Journal of Consulting and Clinical Psychology, 62,* 221–227.

Haldeman, D. C. (2002). Gay rights, patient rights: The implications of sexual orientation conversion therapy. *Professional Psychology: Research and Practice, 33*(3), 260–264.

Halleck, S. L. (1971). *The politics of therapy.* New York: Science House.

Hammen, C. (1999). The emergence of an interpersonal approach to depression. In T. Joiner & J. C. Coyne (Eds.), *The interactional nature of depression* (pp. 21–35). Washington, DC: American Psychological Association.

Hamilton, M. (1959). The assessment of anxiety states by rating. *British Journal of Medical Psychology, 32,* 50–55.

Hancock, K. (1995). Psychotherapy with lesbians and gay men. In A. D'Augelli & C. Patterson (Eds.), *Gay, lesbian and bisexual identities over the lifespan: Psychological perspectives* (pp. 398–432). New York: Oxford University Press.

Hancock, K. A. (2000). Lesbian, gay and bisexual lives: Basic issues in psychotherapy training and practice. In B. Greene & G. L. Croom (Eds.), *Education, research, and practice in lesbian, gay, bisexual, and transgendered psychology: A resource manual.* Thousand Oaks, CA: Sage.

Hatch, M. L., Friedman, S., & Paradis, C. M. (1996). Behavioral treatment of Obsessive–compulsive disorder in African Americans. *Cognitive and Behavioral Practice, 3,* 303–315.

Hayes, S. C. (1993). Analytic goals and the varieties of scientific contextualism. In S. C. Hayes, L. J. Hayes, H. W. Reese, & T. R. Sarbin (Eds.), *Varieties of scientific contextualism* (pp. 11–27). Reno, NV: Context Press.

Hayes, S. C. (2002). Buddhism, and acceptance and commitment therapy. *Cognitive and Behavioral Practice, 9,* 58–66.

Hayes, S. C., Barnes-Holmes, D., & Roche, B. (Eds.). (2001). *Relational frame theory: A post-Skinnerian account of human language and cognition.* New York: Kluwer Academic/Plenum.

Hayes, S. C., & Brownstein, A. J. (1986). Mentalism, behavior-behavior relations, and a behavior analytic view of the purposes of science. *The Behavior Analyst, 9*(2), 175–190.

Hayes, S. C., Hayes, L. J., & Reese, H. W. (1988). Finding the philosophical core: A review of Stephen Pepper's *World Hypotheses. Journal of the Experimental Analysis of Behavior, 50,* 97–111.

Hayes, S. C., Strosahl, K. D., & Wilson, K. G. (1999). *Acceptance and commitment therapy: An experiential approach to behavior change.* New York: Guilford Press.

Hayes, S. C., & Toarmino, D. (1995). If behavioral principles are generally applicable, why is it necessary to understand cultural diversity? *the Behavior Therapist, 18,* 21–23.

Heimberg, R. G., Horner, K. J., Juster, H. R., Safren, S. A., Brown, E. J., Schneier, F. R., & Liebowitz, M. R. (1999). Psychometric properties of the Liebowitz Social Anxiety Scale. *Psychological Medicine, 29,* 199–212.

Heimberg, R. G., Mueller, G., Holt, C. S., Hope, D. A., & Liebowitz, M. R. (1992). Assessment of anxiety in social interaction and being observed by others: The

Social Interaction Anxiety Scale and the Social Phobia Scale. *Behavior Therapy*, 23, 357–368.

Herek, G. M. (1999). AIDS and stigma. *American Behavioral Scientist*, 42, 1106–1116.

Herek, G. M., & Capitanio, J. P. (1999). AIDS stigma and sexual prejudice. *American Behavioral Scientist*, 42, 1130–1147.

Herrell, R., Goldberg, J., True, W. R., Ramakrishnan, V., Lyons, M., Eisen, S., & Tsuang, M. T. (1999). Sexual orientation and suicidality: A co-twin control study in adult men. *Archives of General Psychiatry*, 56, 867–874.

Hersen, M., & Bellack, A. S. (1981). *Behavioral assessment: A practical handbook* (2nd ed.). Elmsford, NY: Pergamon.

Hoge, D. R. (1996). Religion in America: The demographics of belief and affiliation. In E. P. Shafranske (Ed.), *Religion and the clinical practice of psychology* (pp. 21–41). Washington, DC: American Psychological Association.

Hollon, S. D. (2001). Behavioral activation treatment for depression: A commentary. *Clinical Psychology: Science and Practice*, 8, 271–274.

Hooker, E. (1957). The adjustment of the male overt homsexual. *Journal of Projective Techniques*, 21, 18–31.

Hope, D. A., Heimberg, R. G., Juster, H. R., & Turk, C. L. (2000). *Managing social anxiety: A cognitive-behavioral therapy approach client workbook*. San Antonio, TX: TherapyWorks: Psychological Corp.

Hyman, S. M. (2002). The shirtless jock therapist and the bikini-clad client: An exploration of chance extratherapeutic encounters. In A. A. Lazarus & O. Zur (Eds.), *Dual relationships and psychotherapy* (pp. 348–359). New York: Springer.

Isay, R. A. (1991). The homosexual analyst: Clinical considerations. *Psychoanalytic Study of the Child*, 46, 199–216.

Jacobson, N. S. (1989). The politics of intimacy. *the Behavior Therapist*, 12, 29–32.

Jacobson, N. S., & Addis, M. E. (1993). Research on couples and couple therapy: What do we know? Where are we going? *Journal of Consulting and Clinical Psychology*, 61, 85–93.

Jacobson, N. S., & Christensen, A. (1996). *Acceptance and change in couple therapy: A therapists guide to transforming relationships*. New York: Norton.

Jacobson, N. S., Christensen, A. C., Prince, S. E., Cordova, J., & Eldridge, K. (2000). Integrative behavioral couple therapy: An acceptance-based, promising new treatment for couple discord. *Journal of Consulting and Clinical Psychology*, 68, 351–355.

Jacobson, N. S., Dobson, K. Truax, P. A., Addis, M. E., Koerner, K., Gollan, J. K., Gortner, E., & Prince, S. E. (1996). A component analysis of cognitive-behavioral treatment for depression. *Journal of Consulting and Clinical Psychology*, 64, 295–304.

Jacobson, N. S., & Margolin, G. (1979). *Marital therapy: Strategies based on social learning and behavior exchange principles*. New York: Brunner/Mazel.

Jacobson, N. S., Martell, C. R., & Dimidjjian, S. (2001). Behavioral activation treatment for depression: Returning to contextual roots. *Clinical Psychology: Science and Practice*, 8, 255–270.

Jacobson, N. S., Schmaling, K. B., & Holtzworth-Munroe, A. (1987). A component analysis of behavioral marital therapy: Two-year follow-up and prediction of relapse. *Journal of Marital and Family Therapy*, 13, 187–195.

Johnston, S., de Wit, J. B. F., Janssen, M., Coutinho, R. A., & van Griensven, G. J. P. (1999). Do today's young homosexual men practice safer sex than today's older homosexual men did when they were young?: An analysis of sexual behavior change across cohorts in Amsterdam. *AIDS and Behavior, 3*, 75–81.

Jones, M. A., & Gabriel, M. A. (1999). Utilization of psychotherapy by lesbians, gay men, and bisexuals: Findings from a nationwide survey. *American Journal of Orthopsychiatry, 69*, 209–219.

Kagan, J. (1994). *Galen's prophecy*. New York: Basic Books.

Katz, P. A., & Ksansnak, K. R. (1994). Developmental aspects of gender role flexibility and traditionality in middle childhood and adolescence. *Developmental Psychology, 30*, 272–282.

Kauth, M. R., Hartwig, M. J., & Kalichman, S. C. (2000). Health behavior relevant to psychotherapy with lesbian, gay, and bisexual clients. In R. M. Perez, K. A. DeBord, & K. J. Bieschke (Eds.), *Handbook of counseling and psychotherapy with lesbian, gay, and bisexual clients* (pp. 435–456). Washington, DC: American Psychological Association.

Keane, T. M. (1998). Psychological and behavioral treatments of post-traumatic stress disorder. In P. E. Nathan & J. M. Gorman (Eds.), *A guide to treatments that work* (pp. 398–407). Oxford, UK: Oxford University Press.

Keane, T. M., Gerardi, R. J., Quinn, S. J., & Litz, B. T. (1992). Behavioral treatment of post-traumatic stress disorder. In S. M. Turner, K. S. Calhoun, & H. E. Adams (Eds.), *Handbook of clinical behavior therapy* (2nd ed., pp. 87–97). New York: Wiley.

Kessler, R. C., McGonagle, K. A., Zhao, S., Nelson, C. B., Hughes, M., Eshleman, S., Wittchen, H. U., & Kendler, K. S. (1994). Lifetime and 12-month prevalence of DSM-III-R psychiatric disorders in the United States: Results from the National Comorbidity Survey. *Archives of General Psychiatry, 51*, 8–19.

Kilpatrick, D. G., Saunders, B. E., Amick-McMullan, A., Best, C. L., Veronen, L. J., & Resnick, H. S. (1989). Victim and crime factors associated with the development of crime-related post-traumatic stress disorder. *Behavior Therapy, 20*, 199–214.

Kinsey, A. C., Pomeroy, W. B., & Martin, C. E. (1948). *Sexual behavior in the human male*. Philadelphia: Saunders.

Kite, M. E., & Whitley, B. E. Jr. (1998). Do heterosexual wmen and men differ in their attitudes toward homosexuality?: A conceptual and methodological analysis. In G. M. Herek (Ed.), *Stigma and sexual orientation: Understanding prejudice against lesbians, gay men, and bisexuals* (pp. 39–61). Thousand Oaks, CA: Sage.

Kitzinger, C. (1995). Social constructionism: Implications for lesbian and gay psychology. In A. R. D'Augelli & C. J. Patterson (Eds.), *Lesbian, gay, and bisexual identities over the lifespan: Psychological perspectives* (pp. 136–161). New York: Oxford University Press.

Koerner, K., & Dimeff, L. A. (2000). Further data on dialectical behavior therapy. *Clinical Psychology: Science and Practice, 7*, 104–112.

Kohlenberg, R. J. (1974). Treatment of a homosexual pedophiliac using *in vivo* desensitization: A case study. *Journal of Abnormal Psychology, 83*, 192–195.

Kohlenberg, R. J., Kanter, J. W., Bolling, M. Y., Parker, C. R., & Tsai, M. (2002). Enhancing cognitive therapy for depression with functional analytic psychotherapy: Treatment guidelines and empirical findings. *Cognitive and Behavioral Practice, 9*, 213–229.

Kohlenberg, R. J., & Tsai, M. (1991). *Functional analytic psychotherapy: Creating intense and curative therapeutic relationships.* New York: Plenum.

Kohlenberg, R. J., & Tsai, M. (1993). Hidden meaning: A behavioral approach. *the Behavior Therapist, 16*, 80–82.

Kohlenberg, R. J., & Tsai, M. (1994). Improving cognitive therapy for depression with functional analytic psychotherapy: Theory and case study. *The Behavior Analyst, 17*, 305–330.

Kuehlwein, K. T., & Gottschalk, D. I. (2000). Legal and psychological issues confronting lesbian, bisexual, and gay couples and families. In F. W. Kaslow (Ed.), *Handbook of couple and family forensics: A sourcebook for mental health and legal professionals* (pp. 164–187). New York: Wiley.

Kurdek, L. A. (1987). Sex-role schema and psychological adjustment in coupled homosexual and heterosexual men and women. *Sex Roles, 17*, 549–562.

Kurdek, L. A. (1992). Relationship stability and relationship satisfaction in cohabiting gay and lesbian couples: A prospective longitudinal test of the contextual and interdependence models. *Journal of Social and Personal Relationships, 9*, 125–142.

Kurdek, L. A. (1995). Lesbian and gay couples. In R. D'Augelli & C. J. Patterson (Eds.), *Lesbian, gay, and bisexual identities over the lifespan: Psychological perspectives* (pp. 243–261). New York: Oxford University Press.

Kurdek, L. A. (1998). Relationship outcomes and their predictors: Longitudinal evidence from heterosexual married, gay cohabiting, and lesbian cohabiting couples. *Journal of Marriage and the Family, 60*, 553–568.

Kurdek, L. A., & Schmitt, J. P. (1986). Relationship quality of partners in heterosexual married, heterosexual cohabiting, and gay and lesbian relationships. *Journal of Personality and Social Psychology, 51*(4), 711–720.

Lazarus, A. A. (1971). *Behavior therapy and beyond.* New York: McGraw-Hill.

Lazarus, A. A. (1994a). How certain boundaries and ethics diminish therapeutic effectiveness. *Ethics and Behavior, 4*, 255–261.

Lazarus, A. A. (1994b). The illusion of the therapist's power and the patient's fragility: My rejoinder. *Ethics and Behavior, 4*, 299–306.

Lewinsohn, P. M., Youngren, M. A., & Grosscup, S. J. (1979). Reinforcement and depression. In R. A. Depue (Ed.), *The psychobiology of depressive disorders: Implications for the effects of stress* (pp. 291–316). New York: Academic Press.

Liebowitz, M. R. (1987). Social phobia. *Modern Problems in Pharmacopsychiatry, 22*, 141–173.

Linehan, M. M. (1993a). *Cognitive-behavioral treatment of borderline personality disorder.* New York: Guilford Press.

Linehan, M. M. (1993b). *Skills training manual for treating borderline personality disorder.* New York: Guilford Press.

Linehan, M. M. (2000). Commentary on innovations in dialectical behavior therapy. *Cognitive and Behavioral Practice, 7*, 478–480.

Linehan, M. M., Armstrong, H. E., Suarez, A., Allmon, D., & Heard, H. L. (1991). Cognitive-behavioral treatment of chronically parasuicidal borderline patients. *Archives of General Psychiatry, 48*, 1060–1064.

Loftus, E. F. (1980). *Memory: Surprising new insights into how we remember and why we forget.* Reading, MA: Addison-Wesley.

Longres, J. F. (1996). *Men of color: A context for service to homosexually active men.* New York: Harrington Park Press.

Lynch, T. R. (2000). Treatment of elderly depression with personality disorder comorbidity using dialectical behavior therapy. *Cognitive and Behavioral Practice, 7*(3), 468–477.

MacPhillamy, D. J., & Lewinsohn, P. M. (1982). The Pleasant Events Schedule: Studies on reliability, validity and scale inter-correlation. *Journal of Consulting and Clinical Psychology, 50,* 363–380.

Mahoney, M. J. (1995). Theoretical developments in the cognitive and constructive psychotherapies. In M. J. Mahoney (Ed.), *Cognitive and constructive psychotherapies: Theory, research, and practice* (pp. 3–19). New York: Springer.

Malyon, A. K. (1982). Psychotherapeutic implications of internalized homophobia in gay men. In J. C. Gonsiorek (Ed.), *Homosexuality and psychotherapy: A practitioner's handbook of affirmative models* (pp. 59–69). New York: Haworth Press.

Margolin, G., & Weiss, R. L. (1978). Comparative evaluation of therapeutic components associated with behavioral marital treatments. *Journal of Consulting and Clinical Psychology, 46,* 1476–1486.

Marlatt, G. A. (1985). Relapse prevention: Theoretical rationale and overview of the the model. In G. A. Marlatt & J. R. Gordon (Eds.), *Relapse prevention: Maintenance strategies in the treatment of addictive behaviors* (pp. 3–70). New York: Guilford Press.

Marlatt, G. A., & Gordon, J. R. (1985). *Relapse prevention: Maintenance strategies in the treatment of addictive behaviors.* New York: Brunner/Mazel.

Marlatt, G. A., Larimer, M. E., Baer, J. S., & Quigley, L. A. (1993). Harm reduction for alcohol problems: Moving beyond the controlled drinking controversy. *Behavior Therapy, 24,* 461–504.

Marlatt, G. A., Pagano, R. R., Rose, R. M., & Marques, J. K. (1984). Effects of meditation and relaxation training upon alcohol use in male social drinkers. In D. H. Shapiro & R. N. Walsh (Eds.), *Mediation: Classic and contemporary perspectives* (pp. 105–120). New York: Aldine Press.

Marmor, J. (Ed.). (1980). *Homosexual behavior: A modern reappraisal.* New York: Basic Books.

Martell, C. R. (1999). Behavior therapy and sexual minorities: Thoughts on progress and future directions. *the Behavior Therapist, 22,* 194–195.

Martell, C. R. (2001). Including sexual orientation issues in research related to cognitive and behavioral therapies. *the Behavior Therapist, 24,* 214–216.

Martell, C. R., Addis, M. E., & Jacobson, N. S. (2001). *Depression in context: Strategies for guided action.* New York: Norton.

Martell, C. R., & Land, T. E. (2002). Cognitive-behavioral therapy with gay and lesbian couples. In T. Patterson (Ed.), *Comprehensive handbook of psychotherapy: Vol. 2. Cognitive-behavioral approaches* (pp. 451–468). New York: Wiley.

Masten, A. S. (2001). Ordinary magic: Resilience processes in development. *American Psychologist, 56,* 227–238.

Matthews, C. R., & Lease, S. H. (2000). Focus on lesbian, gay, and bisexual families. In R. M. Perez, K. A. DeBord, & K. J. Bierschke (Eds.), *Handbook of counseling and psychotherapy with lesbian, gay and bisexual clients* (pp. 249–273). Washington, DC: American Psychological Association.

Mattick, R. P., & Clarke, J. C. (1998). Development and validation of measures of social phobia scrutiny fear and social interaction anxiety. *Behaviour Research and Therapy, 36,* 455–470.

McCann, R. A., Ball, E. M., & Ivanoff, A. (2000). DBT with an inpatient forensic population: The CMHIP forensic model. *Cognitive and Behavioral Practice, 7*(4), 447–456.

McCullough, J. (2001). *Treatment for chronic depression: Cognitive behavioral analysis system of psychotherapy (CBASP).* New York: Guilford Press.

McLeod, A., & Crawford, I. (1998). The postmodern family: An examination of the psychosocial and legal perspectives of gay and lesbian parenting. In G. M. Herek (Ed.), *Stigma and sexual orientation: Understanding prejudice against lesbians, gay men, and bisexuals* (pp. 211–222). Thousand Oaks, CA: Sage.

McNair, L. D. (1996). African American women and behavior therapy: Integrating theory, culture, and clinical practice. *Cognitive and Behavioral Practice, 3,* 337-349.

McNally , R. J. (2003). Progress and controversy in the study of posttraumatic stress disorder. *Annual Review of Psychology, 54,* 229–252.

McWhirter, D. P., & Mattison, A. M. (1984). *The male couple: How relationships develop.* Englewood Cliffs, NJ: Prentice-Hall.

Menin, D. S., Turk, C. L., & Heimberg, R. G. (2003). Focusing on the regulation of emotion: A new direction for conceptualizing and treating generalized anxiety disorder. In M. A. Reinecke & D. A. Clark (Eds.), *Cognitive therapy over the lifespan: Theory, research and practice* (pp. 60–89). Cambridge: Cambridge University Press.

Meyer, I. H., & Dean, L. (1998). Internalized homophobia, intimacy, and sexual behavior among gay and bisexual men. In G. M. Herek (Ed.), *Stigma, and sexual orientation: Understanding prejudice against lesbians, gay men, and bisexuals: Vol. 2. Psychological perspectives on lesbian and gay issues* (pp. 160–186). Thousand Oaks, CA: Sage.

Meyer, T. J., Miller, M. L., Metzger, R. L., & Borkovec, T. D. (1990). Development and validation of the Penn State Worry Questionnaire. *Behaviour Research and Therapy, 28,* 487–495.

Miller, A. L., & Rathus, J. H. (2000). Introduction to special series: Dialectical behavior therapy: Adaptations and new applications. *Cognitive and Behavioral Practice, 7,* 420–424.

Miller, W. R., & Rollnick, S. (2002). *Motivational interviewing (2nd ed.): Preparing people for change.* New York: Guilford Press.

Mimiaga, M., Berg, M., & Safren, S. A. (2002, November). *Sexual minority men seeking services: A retrospective study of the mental health concerns of men who have sex with men (MSM) in an urban LGBT community health clinic.* Poster presented at the annual meeting of the Association for Advancement of Behavior Therapy, Special Interest Group Poster Session, Reno, NV.

Morganstern, K. P., & Tevlin, H. E. (1981). Behavioral interviewing. In M. Hersen & A. S. Bellack (Eds.), *Behavioral assessment: A practical handbook* (2nd ed., pp. 71–100). Elmsford, NY: Pergamon Press.

Morin, C. M. (1993). *Insomnia: Psychological assessment and management*. New York: Guilford Press.

National Association of Social Workers. (1996). *Code of Ethics of the National Association of Social Workers*. Retrieved October 2, 2000, from *http://www.naswdc.org/pubs/code/default.asp*.

Neimeyer, R. A. (1995). Constructivist psychotherapies: Features, foundations, and future directions. In R. A. Neimeyer & M. J. Mahoney (Eds.), *Constructivism in psychotherapy* (pp. 11–38). Washington, DC: American Psychological Association.

Neimeyer, R. A., & Mahoney, M. J. (1995). *Constructivism in psychotherapy*. Washington, DC: American Psychological Association.

Nelson, R. O., & Hayes, S. C. (1981). Nature of behavioral assessment. In M. Hersen & A. S. Bellack (Eds.), *Behavioral assessment: A practical handbook* (2nd ed., pp. 3–37). Elmsford, NY: Pergamon.

Newman, M. G., & Borkovec, T. D. (1995). Cognitive-behavioral treatment of generalized anxiety disorder. *Clinical Psychologist, 48*, 5–7.

Nezu, A. M., Ronan, G. F., Meadows, E. A., & McClure, K. S. (2000). *Practitioner's guide to empirically based measures of depression*. New York: Kluwer Academic/Plenum.

Nicolosi, J. (1991). *Reparative therapy of male homsexuality: A new clinical Approach*. Northvale, NJ: Jason Aronson.

Nietzel, M. T., & Bernstein, D. A. (1981). Assessment of anxiety and fear. In M. Hersen & A. S. Bellack (Eds.), *Behavioral assessment: A practical handbook* (2nd ed., pp. 215–245). Elmsford, New York: Peramon Press.

Nolen-Hoeksema, S., Morrow, J., & Fredrickson, B. L. (1993). Response styles and the duration of episodes of depressed mood. *Journal of Abnormal Psychology, 102*, 20–28.

Ossana, S. M. (2000). Relationship and couples counseling. In R. M. Perez, K. A. DeBord, & K. J. Bierschke (Eds.), *Handbook of counseling and psychotherapy with lesbian, gay and bisexual clients* (pp. 275–302). Washington, DC: American Psychological Association.

Otto, M. W., & Safren, S. A. (2000). Mechanisms of action in the treatment of social phobia. In S. G. Hofmann, P. M. DiBartolo, & H. R. Juster (Eds.), *Social phobia and social anxiety: An integration* (pp. 391–407). Needham Heights, MA: Allyn & Bacon.

Pakenham, K. I., Dadds, M. R., & Terry, D. J. (1994). Relationships between adjustment to HIV and both social support and coping. *Journal of Consulting and Clinical Psychology, 62*(6), 1194–1203.

Papageorgiou, C., & Wells, A. (2001). Treatment of recurrent major depression with attention training. *Cognitive and Behavioral Practice, 7*, 407–413.

Patterson, C. J. (1995). Sexual orientation and human development: An overview. *Developmental Psychology, 31*, 3–11.

Peplau, L. A., Garnets, L. D., Spalding, L. R., Conley, T. D., & Veniegas, R. C. (1998). A critique of Bem's "Exotic Becomes Erotic" theory of sexual orientation. *Psychological Review, 105*, 387–394.

Pepper, S. C. (1942). *World hypotheses: A study in evidence*. Berkeley: University of California Press.

Perez, R. M., DeBord, K. A., & Bieschke, K. J. (2000). *Handbook of counseling and psy-*

chotherapy with lesbian, gay, and bisexual clients. Washington, DC: American Psychological Association.

Persons, J. B. (1989). *Cognitive therapy in practice: A case formulation approach.* New York: Norton.

Persons, J. B., Burns, D. D., & Perloff, J. M. (1998). Predictors of dropout and outcome in private practice patients treated with cognitive therapy for depression. *Cognitive Therapy and Research, 12,* 557–575.

Persons, J. B., & Davidson, J. (2001). Cognitive-behavioral case formulation. In K. S. Dobson (Ed.), *Handbook of cognitive-behavioral therapies* (2nd ed., pp. 86–110). New York: Guilford Press.

Persons, J. B., Davidson, J., & Tompkins, M. A. (2001). *Essential components of cognitive-behavior therapy for depression.* Washington, DC: American Psychological Association.

Philips, H. C. (1988). *The psychological management of chronic pain: A treatment manual.* New York: Springer.

Phillipson, S. J. (2002). I think it moved: The understanding and treatment of the obsessional doubt related to sexual orientation and relationship substantiation, Part I. *OCD Newsletter, 16,* 4–5, 12.

Pollack M. H., Otto M. W., & Rosenbaum J. F. (Eds.). (1996). *Challenges in clinical practice: Pharmacologic and psychosocial strategies.* New York: Guilford Press.

Purcell, D. W., Campos, P. E., & Perilla, J. L. (1996). Therapy with lesbians and gay men: A cognitive behavioral perspective. *Cognitive and Behavioral Practice, 3*(2), 391–415.

Rapee, R. M., & Heimberg, R. G. (1997). A cognitive-behavioral model of anxiety in social phobia. *Behaviour Research and Therapy, 35,* 741–756.

Rathus, J. H., & Miller, A. L. (2000). Dialectical behavior therapy for adolescents: Dialectical dilemmas and secondary treatment targets. *Cognitive and Behavioral Practice, 7,* 425–434.

Remafedi, G. (1994). The state of knowledge on gay, lesbian, and bisexual youth suicide. In G. Remafedi (Ed.), *Death by denial: Studies of suicide in gay and lesbian teenagers* (pp. 7–14). Boston: Alyson Publishers.

Resick, P. A., Nishith, P., Weaver, T. L., Astin, M. C., & Feuer, C. A. (2002). A comparison of cognitive-processing therapy with prolonged exposure and a waiting condition for the treatment of chronic posttraumatic stress disorder in female rape victims. *Journal of Consulting and Clinical Psychology, 70*(4), 867–879.

Resick, P. A., & Schnicke, M. K. (1992). Cognitive processing therapy for sexual assault victims. *Journal of Consulting and Clinical Psychology, 60,* 748–756.

Reynolds, A. L., & Hanjorgiris, W. F. (2000). Coming out: Lesbian, gay, and bisexual identity development. In R. M. Perez, K. A. DeBord, & K. J. Bieschke (Eds.), *Handbook of counseling and psychotherapy with lesbian, gay, and bisexual clients* (pp. 35–56). Washington, DC: American Psychological Association.

Roberts, L. J., & Marlatt, G. A. (1998). Guidelines for relapse prevention. In G. P. Koocher, J. C. Norcross, & S. S. Hill III (Eds.), *Psychologists' desk reference* (pp. 243–247). New York: Oxford University Press.

Roberts, L. J., & Marlatt, G. A. (1999). Harm reduction. In P. J. Ott, R. E. Tarter, & R. T. Ammerman (Eds.), *Sourcebook on substance abuse: Etiology, epidemiology, and treatment* (pp. 389–398). Boston: Allyn & Bacon.

Robins, C. J. (2002). Zen principles and mindfulness practice in dialectical behavior therapy. *Cognitive and Behavioral Practice, 9,* 50–57.

Roche, B., & Barnes-Holmes, D. (2002). Human sexual arousal: A modern behavioral approach. *The Behavior Analyst Today, 3,* 145–154. Retrieved January 31, 2003, from *http://www.behavior-analyst-online.org.*

Rogers, J. L., Emanuel, K., & Bradford, J. (2003). Sexual minorities seeking services: A retrospective study of the mental health issues of lesbian and bisexual women. *Journal of Lesbian Studies, 1,* 127–146.

Rosen, J. C. (1995). The nature of body dysmorphic disorder and treatment with cognitive behavior therapy. *Cognitive and Behavioral Practice, 2,* 143–166.

Rosen, H., & Kuehlwein, K. T. (1996). *Constructing realities: Meaning-making perspectives for psychotherapists.* San Francisco: Jossey-Bass.

Roszak, T. (2001). *Longevity revolution: As boomers become elders.* Berkeley, CA: Berkeley Hills.

Rothbaum, B. A., & Foa, E. B. (2000). *Reclaiming your life after rape: A cognitive-behavioral therapy for PTSD client workbook.* San Antonio, TX: TherapyWorks: Psychological Corp.

Rotheram-Borus, M. J., & Fernandez, I. (1995). Sexual orientation and developmental challenges experienced by gay and lesbian youths. *Suicide and Life-Threatening Behavior, 25*(Suppl.), 26–33.

Rust, P. (1996). Monogamy and polyamory: Relationship issues for bisexuals. In B. A. Firestein (Ed.), *Bisexuality: The psychology and politics of an invisible minority* (pp. 127–148). Newbury Park, CA: Sage.

Safran, J. D., & Segal, Z. V. (1990). *Interpersonal processes in cognitive therapy.* New York: Jason Aronson.

Safren, S. A., & Heimberg, R. G. (1998). Suicidality in gay, lesbian, and bisexual youth. *the Behavior Therapist, 21,* 147–152.

Safren, S. A., Heimberg, R. G., Brown, E. J., & Holle, C. (1997). Quality of life in patients with social phobia. *Depression and Anxiety, 4,* 126–133.

Safren, S. A., Heimberg, R. G., Horner, K. J., Juster, H. R., Schneier, F. R., & Leibowitz, M. R. (1999). Factor structure of social fears: The Liebowitz Social Anxiety Scale. *Journal of Anxiety Disorders, 13,* 253–270.

Safren, S. A., Heimberg, R. G., & Juster, H. R. (1997). The relationship of patient expectancies to initial severity and treatment outcome in cognitive-behavioral group treatment of social phobia. *Journal of Consulting and Clinical Psychology, 65,* 694–698.

Safren, S. A., Heimberg, R. G., & Turk, C. L. (1998). Factor structure of the Social Interaction Anxiety Scale and the Social Phobia Scale. *Behaviour Research and Therapy, 36*(4), 443–453.

Safren, S. A., Hollander, G., Hart, T. A., & Heimberg, R. G. (2001). Cognitive-behavioral therapy with lesbian, gay, and bisexual youth. *Cognitive and Behavioral Practice, 8,* 215–223.

Safren, S. A., & Pantalone, D. (in press). Social anxiety and barriers to resilience in lesbian, gay, and bisexual adolescents. In A. M. Omoto & H. Kurtzman (Eds.), *Scientific perspectives on sexual orientation, mental health, and substance use.* Washington, DC: American Psychological Association.

Salkovskis, P. M., & Kirk, J. (1996). Obsessional disorders. In K. Hawton, P. M.

Salkovskis, J. Kirk, & D. M. Clark (Eds.), *Cognitive behaviour therapy for psychiatric problems: A practical guide*. Oxford, UK: Oxford University Press.

Sandfort, T. G., de Graaaf, R., Bijl, R., & Schnabel, P. (2001). Same-sex sexual behavior and psychiatric disorders. *Archives of General Psychiatry, 58*, 85–91.

Sarason, B. R., Sarason, I. G., & Pierce, G. R. (1990). *Social supports: An interactional view*. New York: Wiley.

Savin-Williams, R. C. (1990). *Gay and lesbian youth: Expressions of identity*. New York: Hemisphere.

Savin-Williams, R.C. (1994). Verbal and physical abuse as stressors in the lives of lesbian, gay male, and bisexual youths: Associations with school problems, running away, substance use, prostitution, and suicide. *Journal of Consulting and Clinical Psychology, 62*, 261–269.

Savin-Williams, R. C. (2001). Suicide attempts among sexual-minority youths: Population and measurement issues. *Journal of Consulting and Clinical Psychology, 69*, 983–991.

Savin-Williams, R. C., & Cohen, K. M. (1996). Psychosocial outcomes of verbal and physical abuse among lesbian, gay, and bisexual youths. In R. C. Savin-Williams & K. M. Cohen (Eds.), *The lives of lesbians, gays, and bisexuals: Children to adults* (pp. 181–194). Orlando, FL: Harcourt Brace.

Schroeder, M., & Shidlo, A. (2001a, November). *Attempts to change a homosexual orientation: A long-term study of iatrogenic effects of aversion therapies*. Paper presented at the annual meeting of the Association for Advancement of Behavior Therapy, Philadelphia, PA.

Schroeder, M., & Shidlo, A. (2001b). Ethical issues in sexual orientation conversion therapies: An empirical study of consumers. In A. Shidlo, M. Schroeder, & J. Drescher (Eds), *Sexual conversion therapy: Ethical, clinical and research perspectives* (pp. 131–166). New York: Haworth Medical Press.

Schrof, J. M., & Schultz, S. (1999, March 8). Melancholy. *U.S. News & World Report*, pp. 56–63.

Schuyler, D. (1991). *A practical guide to cognitive therapy*. New York: Norton.

Segal, Z. V., Williams, J. M. G., & Teasdale, J. D. (2002). *Mindfulness-based cognitive therapy for depression: A new approach to preventing relapse*. New York: Guilford Press.

Seligman, M. E. P. (1998). *Learned optimism: How to change your mind and your life*. New York: Pocket Books (Simon & Schuster).

Shidlo, A. (1994). Internalized homophobia: Conceptual and empirical issues in measurement. In B. Greene & G. M. Herek (Eds.), *Lesbian and gay psychology: Theory, research, and clinical applications* (pp. 176–205). Thousand Oaks, CA: Sage.

Shidlo, A., & Schroeder, M. (2002). Changing sexual orientation: A consumers' report. *Professional Psychology: Research and Practice, 33*, 249–259.

Siever, M. D. (1994). Sexual orientation and gender as factors in socioculturally acquired vulnerability to body dissatisfaction and eating disorders. *Journal of Consulting and Clinical Psychology, 62*, 252–260.

Skinner, B. F. (1957). *Verbal behavior*. New York: Appleton–Century–Crofts.

Spanier, G. B. (1976). Measuring dyadic adjustment. *Journal of Marriage and the Family, 38*, 15–28.

Spencer, S. B., & Hemmer, R. C. (1993). Therapeutic bias with gay and lesbian clients: A functional analysis. *the Behavior Therapist, 16*, 93–97.

Spring, J. A. (November, 2001). *After the affair: Helping couples rebuild trust and sexual intimacy, and consider forgiveness.* Workshop presented by the Institute for the Advancement of Human Behavior, Seattle, WA.

Stall, R., Mills, T., Williamson, J., Greenword, G., Paul, J., Pollack, L., Binson, D., Osmond, D., & Catania, J. (2002, July). *Co-occurring psychosocial health problems among urban American men who have sex with men are interacting to increase vulnerability to HIV transmission.* Poster presented at the XIV International AIDS Conference, Barcelona, Spain.

Straus, M. A. (1979). Measuring intrafamily conflict and violence: The Conflict Tactics Scale. *Journal of Marriage and the Family, 41*, 75–88.

Straus, M. A., Hamby, S. L., Boney-McCoy, S., & Sugarman, D. B. (1996). The Revised Conflict Tactics Scale (CTS2): Development and preliminary psychometric data. *Journal of Family Issues, 17*(3), 283–316.

Strosahl, K. D., Hayes, S. C., Bergan, J., & Romano, P. (1998). Assessing the field effectiveness of acceptance and commitment therapy: An example of the manipulated training research method. *Behavior Therapy, 29*, 35–64.

Suinn, R. (1990). *Anxiety management training: A behavior therapy.* New York: Plenum Press.

Tafoya, T. (1992). Native gay and lesbian issues: The two-spirited. In B. Berzon (Ed.), *Positively gay* (pp. 342–358). Berkeley, CA: Celestial Arts.

Tafoya, T., & Wirth, D. A. (1996). Native American two-spirit men. In J. F. Longres (Ed.), *Men of color: A context for service to homosexually active men* (pp. 51–67). New York: Harrington Park Press.

Tanaka-Matsumi, J., Seiden, D. Y., & Lam, K. N. (1996). The culturally informed functional assessment interview (CIFA): A strategy for cross-cultural behavioral practice. *Cognitive and Behavioral Practice, 3*, 215–233.

Taub, J. (1999). Bisexual women and beauty norms: A qualitative examination. *Journal of Lesbian Studies, 3*, 27–36.

Taylor, S. E., & Aspinwall, L. G. (1990). Psychosocial aspects of chronic illness. In P. T. Costa Jr. & G. R. Van den Bos (Eds.), *Psychological aspects of serious illness: Chronic conditions, fatal diseases, and clinical care* (pp. 3–60). Washington, DC: American Psychological Association.

Throckmorton, W. (2002). Initial empirical and clinical findings concerning the change process for ex-gays. *Professional Psychology: Research and Practice, 33*, 242–248.

Turkat, I. E. (1985). *Behavioral case formulation.* New York: Plenum Press.

Turner, R. M. (2000). Naturalistic evaluation of dialectical behavior therapy-oriented treatment for borderline personality disorder. *Cognitive and Behavioral Practice, 7*, 413–419.

Valenstein, E. S. (1998). *Blaming the brain: The truth about drugs and mental health.* New York: Free Press.

Watson, D., & Friend, R. (1969). Measurement of social-evaluative anxiety. *Journal of Consulting and Clinical Psychology, 33*, 448–457.

Watzlawick, P. (1996). The construction of clinical "realities." In H. Rosen & K. T.

Kuehlwein (Eds.), *Constructing realities: Meaning-making perspectives for psychotherapists*. San Francisco: Jossey-Bass.

Weiss, R. L., & Cerreto, M. C. (1980). The Marital Status Inventory: Development of a measure of dissolution potential. *American Journal of Family Therapy, 8,* 80–85.

Wells, A. (1990). Panic disorder in association with relaxation-induced anxiety: An attentional training approach to treatment. *Behavior Therapy, 21,* 273–280.

Williams, M. H. (1997). Boundary violations: Do some contended standards of care fail to encompass commonplace procedures of humanistic, behavioral, and eclectic psychotherapies. *Psychotherapy, 34,* 238–249.

Wolpe, J. (1982). *The practice of behavior therapy* (3rd ed.). Elmsford, NY: Pergamon.

Yarhouse, M. A. (1998). Group therapies for homosexuals seeking change. *Journal of Psychology and Theology, 26,* 247–258.

Yarhouse, M. A., & Burkett, L. A. (2002). An inclusive response to LGB and conservative religious persons: The case of same-sex attraction and behavior. *Professional Psychology: Research and Practice, 33,* 235–241.

Zamora-Hernández, C. E., & Patterson, D. G. (1996). Homosexually active Latino men: Issues for social work practice. In J. F. Longres (Ed.), *Men of color: A context for service to homosexually active men* (pp. 69–91). New York: Harrington Park Press.

Zettle, R. D., & Raines, J. C. (1989). Group cognitive and contextual therapies in treatment of depression. *Journal of Clinical Pychology, 45,* 438–445.

Zinbarg, R. E., Craske, M. G., Barlow, D. H., & O'Leary, T. (1993). *Mastery of your anxiety and worry*. San Antonio, TX: TherapyWorks: Psychological Corp.

Zur, O. (2001). Out-of-office experience: When crossing office boundaries and engaging in dual relationships are clinically beneficial and ethically sound. *Independent Practitioner, 21,* 96–100.

Zur, O., & Lazarus, A. A. (2002). Six arguments against dual relationships and their rebuttals. In A. A. Lazarus & O. Zur (Eds.), *Dual relationships and psychotherapy* (pp. 3–24). New York: Springer.

Index

"f" indicates a figure; "t" indicates a table; "n" indicates a note

255